Praise for *Getting Healthy*

'As a food writer who is particularly interested in mental health and environment too, I've long been a fan of Dr Jenny Goodman. I think we all know now in 2024 that everything is connected, but where and how do we start in actually improving our health and the planet's? And in a long-term, sustainable way? HELP! Dr Jenny is back again with her second book – packed to the brim with her medical experience, her fantastic way with words, her empowering practical tips and the scientific research to back it all up.'

Melissa Hemsley, chef and author of *Real Healthy*

'Dr Jenny Goodman's new book is a treasure! It should be required reading in all high schools. The author has first-hand knowledge of her subject matter. Lots of great advice on how to avoid toxic exposures and what to do to restore health once they've made you ill while eschewing pharmaceutical drugs. The science is highly accurate but not too technical for the lay public. The book is sprinkled with engaging stories of specific cases and is so timely in this age of pervasive toxic chemicals in our food, water and air.'

Stephanie Seneff, PhD, author of *Toxic Legacy*

'Dr Jenny Goodman has a rare ability to communicate complex science in the most easily digestible way. Despite the alarming nature of the subject matter, *Getting Healthy in Toxic Times* is an easy and compelling read. Dr Goodman tackles what is arguably the most pressing issue we face as humans: the damage we have inflicted on our environment and the inevitable harvest of suffering we are now reaping. At the heart of the message she wants to convey to the public is the appreciation of our utter inseparability from nature, of the fact that we are nature and that damaging our environment is an act of self-harm.

In the interests of our well-being, Dr Goodman tackles multiple thorny issues head-on, bringing a wholesome mix of science and humanity to bear on a situation that she finds simply too urgent to mince her words. This book contains a mass of invaluable information collected together to provide a comprehensive resource to protect the health of our and our family's health and well-being, and thereby to contribute to the well-being of our environment and all the other people and species depending on it.

Getting Healthy in Toxic Times needed to be written and Dr Jenny Goodman was ideally placed to have been its author. Now it needs and deserves to be widely read.'

Robin Daly, founder and chairman of Yes to Life,
the UK's integrative cancer care charity

'*Getting Healthy in Toxic Times* is an important book. It shows what humanity is doing to their own environments and to the whole planet, damaging the health of every form of life on earth. Small improvements have been made here and there, but the whole situation is getting worse day by day. In order to make a real difference, we need to think of the root cause of all of this and address that root cause. Is it human greed? Is it the ever-increasing tyranny of global corporations? Is it money-based, merry-go-round "economy"? Is it the modern religion of "individualism" and "looking after number one"? The toxicity of our environment is connected to all other aspects of our lives. To address the environment, we must change as individual human beings and as humanity as a whole. We must become kinder and more loving to everything alive around us and we must get closer to nature.'

Dr Natasha Campbell-McBride, MD, the creator of
the GAPS concept and the GAPS Diet

GETTING HEALTHY
IN TOXIC TIMES

GETTING HEALTHY IN TOXIC TIMES

An ecological doctor's prescription for healing your body and the planet

Dr Jenny Goodman

Chelsea Green Publishing
London, UK
White River Junction, Vermont USA

Commissioning Editor: Muna Reyal
Project Manager: Susan Pegg
Copy Editor: Susan Pegg
Proofreader: Jacqui Lewis
Indexer: MFE Editorial Services
Page Layout: Laura Jones-Rivera

Printed and bound in Great Britain by TJ Books Limited, Padstow, Cornwall.
First printing May 2024.
10 9 8 7 6 5 4 3 2 1 24 25 26 27 28

ISBN 978-1-915294-33-3 (paperback)
ISBN 978-1-915294-34-0 (ebook)
ISBN 978-1-915294-35-7 (audiobook)

Our Commitment to Green Publishing
Chelsea Green sees publishing as a tool for cultural change and ecological stewardship. We strive to align our book manufacturing practices with our editorial mission and to reduce the impact of our business enterprise in the environment. We print our books using vegetable-based inks whenever possible. This book may cost slightly more because it was printed on paper from responsibly managed forests, and we hope you'll agree that it's worth it. *Getting Healthy in Toxic Times* was printed on paper supplied by TJ Books Limited that is certified by the Forest Stewardship Council.

Chelsea Green Publishing
London, UK
White River Junction, Vermont USA
www.chelseagreen.co.uk

Disclaimer: This book is designed to provide helpful information on the subjects discussed. It is not meant to be used, nor should it be used, to diagnose or treat any medical condition. For diagnosis or treatment of any medical problem, please consult your own physician or a suitable professional practitioner. The publisher and author are not liable for any damages or negative consequences from any treatment, action, application or preparation to any person reading or following the information in this book. References are provided for informational purposes only and do not constitute endorsement of any websites or sources. Readers should be aware that the websites listed in this book may change. The information and references included are up to date at the time of writing but given that medical evidence progresses, they may not be up to date at the time of reading. All personal names given in case histories have been changed to preserve privacy/anonymity.

In loving memory of some friends who died before their time:

Stephen Walsh
Helen Rose
Ziva Weaver
Zelda Alexander
Nina Maraney
Geela Caiden
Brian Taylor
Mervyn Lebor
Rose Rose
and
Nickie Shapero (2 October 1957–17 February 1979)

CONTENTS

INTRODUCTION

EVERYTHING IS CONNECTED

Our health and that of the planet are inextricably linked. These days, many of us are concerned about the environment, and many of us are also worrying about the sickness of a beloved relative or friend, or indeed of our own bodies. But we may not have realised that the two concerns are closely connected.

Good medical practice requires thinking about the underlying causes of illness and, as a physician, I have spent decades seeing the direct effects of environmental pollution on people's health. We all know now that nutrition, exercise, relaxation and sleep are crucial determinants of our health, but very little has been written, outside of learned journals, about the devastating impact that pollution is having on our bodies. The purpose of this book is to close that gap, to translate the relevant science into ordinary English, and to demonstrate how pollutants get into us, how they make us sick and how we can avoid them as individuals and, collectively, stop them at source. There is so much we can do improve our health and that of our children, once we become aware of the numerous preventable sources of environmental toxicity. And everything we do to help ourselves will help planet Earth as well; the pollution that is damaging us is equally damaging our wildlife, from monkeys to mosses, butterflies to corals to oak trees.

Do you know, or have you ever known, a person with cancer? That's a question I often ask a room full of people when I'm giving a talk. Usually, almost every hand in the room goes up. This is profoundly shocking, but we have got used to it; cancer has become familiar, normalised, normal. One in two of us, we are told now, will be diagnosed with it. But if I had asked that question of a room full of a hundred comparable people, say, fifty years ago, maybe twenty hands would have gone up. A century ago, perhaps five or six hands. Two hundred years ago, maybe one hand, or none. It's really hard for us to notice that which has become ordinary. Ecologists call this the 'shifting baseline syndrome',[1] meaning that we can only compare the state of today's wildlife – or human health – with what we remember of the past, and that cannot be longer ago than our own lifespan.

It's not just cancer; the situation is similar with other degenerative diseases. Alzheimer's, Parkinson's, multiple sclerosis, diabetes, autism, arthritis, asthma, heart disease, mental illness and infertility are all increasing at astonishing rates. In the UK we have three million people with diabetes, mostly type 2 diabetes, which used to be called 'mature onset diabetes', but now we are seeing it in younger and younger people, even in children. One in three of us suffer from heart disease; nearly a million have dementia in Britain alone.

I have argued in my first book, *Staying Alive in Toxic Times: A Seasonal Guide to Lifelong Health*,[2] (henceforth referred to as *SAITT*) that this dramatic increase is not, contrary to what we are often told, anything to do with ageing. Cancer rates are going up fastest among children. And we are not, in fact, living significantly longer than previous generations, we are just living sicker,[3] with our last years becoming a prolonged twilight of disability and suffering. Yet it should be possible for all of us to live a full, healthy life, eventually dying peacefully, simply of old age. This is not an unreasonable aspiration; it is our birthright.

Our genes only change very, very slowly, over aeons. The vast majority of people suffering today with a chronic, degenerative disease such as Alzheimer's did not have an ancestor with that disease. The sheer speed with which chronic degenerative diseases have increased, over just a very few generations, tells us clearly that we are dealing with environmental, not genetic, factors. It's our environment that has changed so rapidly that the forces of biological evolution just can't keep up. As the *Lancet* Commission on pollution and health said: 'Pollution is the largest environmental cause of disease and death in the world today.'[4]

What's Got into You?

When I first started researching this book, I went into a large bookshop in central London that has many floors. 'Health' was on one floor, 'Environment' on another. ('Health' and 'Medicine' were also on different floors;

that's another story.) But we have to join these dots: whatever's in the air, it's in your lungs and in your bloodstream. Whatever gets into the water: you're drinking it. Whatever is sprayed on the soil: it's in the crops and in the food on your plate. Whichever nutrients are missing from the soil after years of intensive farming: they're missing from your dinner. (What farmers do, I predict, will affect our health more profoundly than anything doctors do.)

So, we have a health crisis and we have an environmental crisis; the roots of the two problems are the same, and the solutions are the same. The causes of our frightening epidemic illnesses are not unknown. As I shall show in this book, we are eating the causes, we are drinking the causes, we are inhaling the causes and some of us are rubbing the causes into our skin. Industrialised agriculture and the petrochemical industry are damaging our nutrition and poisoning our atmosphere, our rivers, our oceans and our soil, and therefore our bodies. We are not and can never be separate from our mother the earth; when we pollute the planet, we pollute ourselves. But it is possible to stop doing both, to heal ourselves and the earth, and this book explains how.

On a small scale, I have seen this work in my practice of ecological medicine, as have my colleagues. We identify the environmental and nutritional roots of a person's illness and enable them to recover by changing several elements of the way they live, including what they eat, what they drink, what's in their home and what they put on their skin. (What they inhale outdoors is of course harder to change; if they live on a polluted main road the solutions are mostly collective and political rather than individual – but we'll come to that in chapter 4.) In making these changes to benefit their own health, people are contributing to the health of the planet too. Here we see an example in the case of 'Ellie'. (In all the case histories in this book, the identity of the patient has been disguised, and their story used with their or their parent's permission.)

ELLIE'S STORY

An eight-month-old baby was brought to see me, covered in eczema. I'll call her Ellie. Her skin was red, raw, sore, even bleeding in places. Her hands were encased in little white cotton mittens to stop her scratching.

Her mum was covering her in a moisturising cream, prescribed by the GP, several times a day. I got out my magnifying glass and read the ingredients list on the pack: paraffin (two types), parabens (two types) and a few other nasties. These are petrochemicals, cheap by-products derived from crude oil. Some of them are potentially carcinogenic, and they also pose a serious fire risk.[5] And the cream wasn't even working. But what alternatives were there? Plenty.

We found out the cause of the eczema – her mum was eating several foods to which Ellie was reacting allergically. (Details of how to do this kind of nutritional detective work are in *SAITT*.) Ellie's mum altered her diet, breastfeeding proceeded more smoothly than before, and the tummy ache and irritability that had also bothered Ellie disappeared as well. Her skin cleared up within a few weeks. Occasionally, Ellie's mum forgets or slips up with her diet, so Ellie gets a flare-up, but her mum now uses a totally natural, herbal cream from a good health food shop; she checks that there are no petrochemicals in the ingredients list. (There are numerous herbs that help with eczema, including chickweed, chamomile, calendula, liquorice root, marshmallow, burdock and evening primrose.)

What has Ellie's skin cream got to do with the state of the planet? A lot. Each time we buy a tube of such paraffin-based cream, whether medicinal or cosmetic – and this stuff is in every chemist's shop – we are supporting an industry that is devastating the earth. Wherever they extract crude oil from beneath the ground, you can't live there, you can't farm there, nothing will grow. The soil and the rivers are poisoned. Ogoniland in Nigeria is the best-known example of a huge area where drilling for oil wrecked the land, and the livelihoods and the lives of the inhabitants. The crude oil that these companies extract goes to make diesel, petrol, plastics and pharmaceuticals like Ellie's skin cream, releasing greenhouse gases in the process. Learning to use natural, nutritional and herbal solutions to health problems like Ellie's eczema is not only better for the patient, it's better for the earth – one fewer purchase of a product that was toxic to the place and people where it was dug up and is eventually toxic to the end user too.

Most serious illness is multifactorial: it has several contributing components rather than just one cause. In ecological medicine, we talk about a person's 'total load'. That 'load' may include injury, infection, stress, assorted nutritional deficiencies and numerous environmental toxins. In treating a sick person, we need to identify these causal components and reduce each of them as much as possible, to lower the total load. The focus in this book is on environmental toxins – pollution – but in practice it isn't often found in isolation. So, in the following case history, we will meet 'Ricky', whose illness resulted primarily from two particular types of environmental toxin, but with lots of other factors, both environmental and nutritional, in the mix.

RICKY'S STORY

Ricky had been suffering from numbness and pain in his hands and feet, severe headaches, fatigue and increasingly blurred vision, for about four months. He had become unable to work because of the headaches, and unable to drive because of the blurred vision. Naturally, he went to an optician, who looked worried and immediately referred him to a neurologist. A brain scan resulted in a diagnosis of multiple sclerosis (MS). Remarkably, he came to see me straight after that; it is far more common for patients to go through the mill of conventional treatment and suffer numerous side effects for many years, with little clinical improvement, before finally consulting a holistic practitioner as a last resort. The fact that Ricky came to see me only four months after his symptoms began is one of the reasons his treatment has been so successful.

I always begin by looking for causes, and in this case we were able to identify the episode that had sparked off the symptoms. Three or four weeks before the symptoms began, Ricky had had his office, where he worked in southern Spain, sprayed for an infestation of cockroaches. The spraying technicians, who wore full protective gear, had warned him not to go near the office for at least forty-eight hours. However, Ricky had important work to do and went into his office shortly after the spraying ended; he spent that day and the following days working there. Within a few short weeks, his MS began.

However, a serious illness like MS usually has many contributing factors; I suspected that the recent insecticide spraying was only the final trigger. We identified a lot of other factors that would have predisposed him to get ill: he had many metal amalgam fillings in his mouth, which contain the neurotoxin mercury. He ate a lot of tuna – up to two tins daily, for a quick lunch – that's more mercury. (We will learn a lot about mercury in chapter 2: where it comes from, how it gets into us, what it does to us, and how to get rid of it and thenceforth avoid it.)

Ricky used a lot of artificial sweeteners as well as sugar, ate no healthy fats, held his mobile phone to his head for many hours a day, slept very little ('too busy'), had several nutrient deficiencies, including the crucial vitamin D, vitamin E, zinc and iodine, and he had additional chemical exposure from frequent flying. This last effect is increasingly referred to as 'aerotoxic syndrome', and it affects pilots and cabin crew even more than frequent flyers; it is described in more detail, with a case history, on pages 263–270 of *SAITT*. Significantly, Ricky had also had a previous insecticide exposure when his attic at home was sprayed for wasps' nests some years before. He had high fluoride levels too; we'll find out where that comes from, what it does to us and what to do about it in chapter 3.

When Ricky came to see me, he had already put himself on Terry Wahls' excellent diet for MS. However, I find it a little too strict for most people, so I added in eggs (organic and free range, of course), good-quality, cold-pressed, organic vegetable oils (as salad dressing, always unheated) and avocados, and focused on removing the vast amounts of refined carbohydrates and artificial additives from Ricky's diet. These had, of course, been another contributing factor. This was really hard for him – it still is – but he mostly sticks to it. When he doesn't, his symptoms return at once, which tells him the diet is working; lapses can be useful! Advanced tests showed that Ricky's mitochondria, the energy-producing organelles in our cells, were not working well, so I gave him what mitochondria need most: magnesium, coenzyme Q10 (CoQ10), carnitine and B vitamins.

On testing, I found two different insecticides in Ricky's system, not surprisingly, and also mercury and cadmium – both neurotoxic metals.

Some of the mercury was actually attached to the gene that makes the myelin protein. This is highly significant; myelin is the fatty insulation that coats and protects the nerves, allowing messages to travel between brain and body. It deteriorates in MS – that's why Ricky's hands and feet had gone numb and his eyesight had become blurred – and repairing it is crucial to recovery. It has a protein component as well as a fatty component, and the protein component is the part that the immune system attacks in people with MS. Multiple sclerosis is an example of an autoimmune disease, and autoimmunity is like beating yourself up at the cellular level.

Now, the immune system is very smart; it has kept us humans alive for hundreds of thousands of years by successfully defending us against invading microbes. (Most Europeans, Asians and North Africans today are descended from people who survived the Black Death, while countless others around them died.) So, the key question is: why would our very clever immune system start attacking the tissues of its own body? This is a question that orthodox medicine does not ask; it just zaps the immune system with steroids to try to make it stop. However, there is good reason to suspect that toxic metals like mercury distort the protein's structure, making it look alien to the immune system's patrolling white blood cells, which then treat it as they would an invading microbe: they destroy it. Furthermore, insecticides are fat-soluble poisons, so they make a beeline for fatty tissues in the body, such as the myelin sheath of the nerves of the central nervous system.

So, my focus was on getting all the toxins out of Ricky's system, to give his myelin a chance to normalise. As well as correcting his nutritional deficiencies, I instituted a detoxification programme for him: very high-dose vitamin C for a few months (as described on page 305 of *SAITT*); glutathione (essential for detox – we do make it ourselves, but some of us, including Ricky, are less able to make it, for genetic reasons); phosphatidyl choline (PC) liquid for getting rid of fat-soluble toxins like insecticides; Epsom salts baths (Epsom salts are magnesium sulphate, and assist with certain of the liver's detox pathways as well as relaxing the muscles); and, most vital of all, organic vegetable juicing every day (described on page 298 of *SAITT*).

After a few months, on my principle of 'put the good stuff in before you take the bad stuff out', Ricky had all his mercury amalgam fillings removed by a super-safe dentist, using the protocols of the International Academy for Oral Medicine and Toxicology (IAOMT) to prevent further release of mercury into the system. He bought a water filter, at my request, so he wasn't drinking chlorine or any of the other tap water contaminants we'll discover in chapter 3. Finally, we moved on to two more detox modalities, saunas and colonic hydrotherapy (explained in chapter 7 of *SAITT*), and I made him promise to avoid all kinds of pesticides forever; this includes eating organic, strictly and permanently. By the end of chapter 1, you will understand why this is so vital.

At the third consultation, a few months after his first visit, Ricky's energy level and vision were substantially improved, sensation was returning to the numb patches on his hands and feet, and he was sleeping normal hours. Re-testing showed that the toxic metals and insecticides were almost gone – and they are now completely gone. By the fourth consult, his eyesight had normalised, to the delight and puzzlement of the optician. The headaches have vanished, and he is essentially back to his former self. BUT if he stops the good oils or the PC liquid, or he goes back to eating sugar or refined carbs, he gets ill again – numbness, weakness, pain. Once back on the regime, he recovers within two weeks. Natural medicine works, especially if started very early on in an illness. But it is hard work: it takes dedication from the patient and support and encouragement from those around him or her; luckily, Ricky has these in plenty.

Good Stuff In, Bad Stuff Out

As you can see from Ricky's story, getting better is not about EITHER improving nutrition OR detoxing pollutants – it's always BOTH. But there are already countless books out there on nutrition, including my own, and that's why it is now time to focus on the Bad Stuff that's making us ill in vast numbers: toxic environmental pollution.

The problem with 'vast numbers', however, is that they're hard to relate to. When it's *your* sister who's got lung cancer, *your* dad who has just been diagnosed with dementia or *your* child who is (God forbid) going through the ordeal of chemo, how can you possibly focus on the Bigger Picture? It's quite natural to put all your energies into the person you love, just doing everything you can to ease the path of that one beloved person. Yet it's likely that there are thousands of families going through the exact same misery at the same time. The cold, dry statistics that are so hard to relate to nevertheless tell the story of these tragedies, multiplied a thousandfold, a millionfold.

The very essence of tragedy is that it is preventable: it didn't need to happen. The purpose of this book is the prevention of such tragedies, through understanding and action. But I recognise that the last thing you can bear to hear, if someone you love dearly is dying too soon or losing their capacity to feed themselves / talk / walk / dance / live freely is that it didn't need to happen. Therefore, it is all the more incumbent upon those of us who are alive, well, still thinking clearly and not currently immersed in nursing a beloved spouse / child / sibling / parent / friend to learn all we can about the causes of these multiple tragedies, the causes I demonstrate in this book. Beyond the dry (but overwhelming) statistics is human pain and, if we clean up our act and clean up our planet, I believe many, if not most, of these tragedies can indeed be prevented. It's not too late.

It may be tempting to put our heads in the sand; but if we can face up to these problems, and acknowledge that they exist, then we can solve them.

How Well Is Our Environment?

In the chapters that follow, I'm going to discuss pollution as it affects us in the different realms of earth, water and air – but of course, they are not really separate realms at all. Air pollution from car fumes, for instance, includes particulate matter: tiny solid particles that fall through the air and land on the earth. They also land on the fruit and vegetables displayed outside the shop on a busy main road. Toxic chemicals discharged into rivers and lakes find their way onto the land as well as into the sea. Conversely, pesticides sprayed onto fields of growing crops find their way into the water table. So do synthetic fertilisers, with disastrous consequences that we'll come across in chapter 1. As regards the Fire chapters, I'm using the term semi-metaphorically; it's about physical rather than chemical pollution: energy in the form of radiation. There is good light and bad light, as we'll see.

The whole planet is one joined-up ecosystem, with everything interconnected, just as the human body is. But just as, when teaching anatomy and physiology, one has to describe the body 'system by system' – for example, the gut and then the circulation, and then the lungs, and so on – while knowing full well that it's all one (and that the interactions between systems are of key importance), so I need to divide up the topic of pollution somehow, to make it possible for us to get our heads around it. And I decided against classifying toxins according to their molecular structure – you'd need a degree in chemistry to make sense of that, and even then it would be tough!

So, forgive me if there seems to be a certain artificiality in these divisions. On the other hand, the categories of Earth, Water, Air and Fire go back many millennia in our shared intellectual history; they're part of our heritage. And they make sense as much in the world of physics as in the worlds of folklore, myth and mysticism.

After Earth, Water, Air and Fire, there is a short chapter about the surprising poisonings of everyday life – what's affecting you in your own home. Indoor pollution is incredibly important yet remarkably easy to get rid of – once you know it's there. In Appendix I, there is a brief look at our mental health, which is being as profoundly affected by environmental pollution as is physical health; the brain is part of the body, after all. Appendix II gives a tiny sample of the industrial pollution episodes that have profoundly affected the health of local communities.

In each chapter, I suggest changes you can make to improve your own health (and that of planet Earth), but please don't feel you have to make all the changes at once! Take your time, absorb the information at your own pace and know that any change you make will make a difference.

This book is about solutions to pollution as much as pollution itself. And in most sections, I'll have to outline the problems before I can begin to look at the existing and potential answers. However, in chapter 1, I'm actually going to start with some of the major solutions because they are centrally important, life-enhancing and already happening. So – let's get down to earth.

CHAPTER ONE

EARTH I: NOURISHING OR TOXIC?

Whatever befalls the earth, befalls the children of the earth.

Ted Perry, *Home*

The soil is alive. It is teeming with creatures, from earthworms to insects to microscopic bacteria and fungi. They form a team, busily interacting with each other and the growing plants and the mineral structure of the soil, to keep it healthy, resilient and fertile. It's buzzing down there! The technical term 'biodiversity' doesn't really light my fire; I'd rather call it 'abundant life, infinite variety'. Here's how it works, and how it keeps us alive and well.

Welcome to the Earth

We need nourishment directly from the plants that we eat, or indirectly from animals that have eaten those plants. Plants take up nutrient minerals from the soil – but it's not as simple as that. The plants need helpers to get those nutrients in. The helpers are called mycorrhizae, tiny filamentous fungi, which attach to the plants' roots. They are so closely attached that they are almost one organism with the plant. In return for the vital minerals that the fungi transfer into the plants' roots, the plants transfer some of the sugars and amino acids that they've made into the fungi. It's called symbiosis: literally 'together living' – essentially, 'you scratch my back, I'll scratch yours', a type of cooperation that occurs more frequently in nature than the fierce competition we hear so much about.

Plants need nitrogen as well as minerals. Well, that shouldn't be a problem; the air around us is 78 per cent nitrogen, so there's no shortage. But hang on – plants can't absorb nitrogen directly from the air, any more than we can. This is where another set of helpers come in: the soil bacteria. These microbes can 'fix' nitrogen into plants, enabling them to absorb and utilise it. The legume family, when they have the right microbes attached, are particularly good at this nitrogen-fixing business; they include peas, beans, lentils, peanuts, clover, vetch and alfalfa. That's why regenerative farmers use these plants frequently, in rotation between the 'cash' crops, to replenish the soil's fertility in a safe and natural way.

Happy soil is also full of earthworms, who go up and down, aerating and oxygenating the earth, stabilising the soil structure so that it is light and crumbly and can absorb rainwater, therefore being less at risk of water run-off and erosion. This enables it to withstand both drought and floods; indeed, it helps to prevent flooding. The worms take nutritious organic matter down from the surface to the deeper layers. They eat dead leaves and other debris, pooing them out transformed into natural fertiliser. Darwin said of earthworms: 'It may be doubted whether there are many other animals that have played so important a part in the history of the world.'

Larger animals too, like cows and sheep and even chickens, do a valuable job of fertilising the earth, returning carbon and nitrogen to the soil. They also stimulate the growth of grass by eating it. As David Attenborough said in the BBC series *Wild Isles*, 'If grasslands are to be rich and diverse, they have to be grazed.'

Healthy, living soil, undisturbed by heavy machinery and free of toxic pesticides and synthetic fertilisers, produces healthy, vibrant food,[1] which makes healthy people – and smarter children.[2] When a farm contains a rich variety of organisms, from bacteria and fungi to plants and animals all living together much as they do in nature, the food that farm produces leads directly to similar biodiversity in our own digestive tracts: a rich and healthy microbiome. This means friendly bacteria and other microbes living symbiotically in our gut, manufacturing essential vitamins and short-chain fatty acids for us, supporting our immune system and our brain function, and enabling us to digest our food properly, leading to maximal physical health and mental clarity. (This is assuming we don't blow it by overdosing on sugar, which feeds all the wrong bugs, or on antibiotics, which destroy the good ones, or on the contraceptive pill or HRT, which encourage overgrowth of yeasts!)

There are many labels currently in use for the kind of soil-friendly, people-friendly agriculture I'm going to describe. Colin Tudge calls it 'enlightened agriculture'.[3] You'll also hear the terms 'regenerative', 'organic', 'no-till', 'permaculture', 'sustainable', 'biodynamic', 'holistic' and 'conservation agriculture', as well as 'agroecology'. There are differences, and the very best farmers fit most or all of these labels, but let's not get too hung up on terminology. They're all going in the right direction. Food from such farms should be uncontaminated by artificial chemicals and rich in nutrients we need because regenerative farming practices continually return nourishment to the soil (whereas conventional intensive farming continually drains them all away). All this is not just in an ideal world but is happening for real on the many regenerative farms now springing up around the UK, some of which I've had the privilege of visiting.

Down on the Farm

Peter Greig welcomes me warmly onto his beautiful farm, Pipers Farm, in Devon. His father, he tells me, was one of the first intensive chicken farmers (broilers, crammed in tight; not free to peck and wander around on the grass) but Peter and his wife Henri have chosen to go in completely the opposite direction.

I have done my homework before I arrive, so I believe I have understood the essential ideas and practices of regenerative farming. I've summarised them below as seven basic principles, along with examples from some of the lovely farms I have visited. The principles are:

1. Farm without pesticides – this means farming organically.
2. Maximise diversity (of plant life).
3. Use cover crops.
4. Conserve the soil structure.
5. Agroforestry – include trees on the farm.
6. Farm without synthetic fertilisers – this is part of being organic too.
7. Integrate animals, naturally pastured.

On Peter's farm, I get to see these principles in action; we'll return to them at intervals in the sections that follow.

1. Farm without Pesticides

Why farm without pesticides? The commonest pesticides in use today, the organophosphates (OPs), are chemicals developed from nerve gases used by the Nazis in the Second World War.[4] They don't just kill their target pests. They kill vital soil microbes[5] and cumulatively they poison whichever animal (human or otherwise) eats the crops they've been sprayed on.[6] After a while, though, pesticides stop working on their target pests; bugs develop resistance to pesticides just as they do to antibiotics. So, then the farmer tries another, and another, and more of the same. Some pesticides end up killing the useful creatures that would naturally prey on the pests. Pesticides do so many different types of damage to our bodies, it's hard to know where to begin. They were designed as nerve poisons, so let's start with what they do to our brain and nervous system.

The OP pesticides interfere with nerve signalling by destroying a vital enzyme, acetylcholinesterase, in the synapse (tiny gap) between two nerve cells. This enzyme has the job of breaking down the neurotransmitter chemical acetylcholine, which transmits the impulse from one nerve cell to the next. Nerve signalling is meant to be an 'on–off' affair: as soon as an impulse has passed down a nerve cell, that cell becomes 'refractory' for a split second; it has a rest and can't respond to subsequent impulses till that split second is over. This rest, though, is only made possible by the enzyme, acetylcholinesterase, doing its job. (The suffix '-ase' tells you it's an enzyme whose particular job is to break a large molecule down into smaller components.)

Pesticides bind tightly to acetylcholinesterase and disable it – they are cholinesterase inhibitors.[7] This leads to nerve cells being stuck in the 'on' mode, resulting in an overload and eventually paralysis of the nerve signalling system. This is one of the most important ways in which pesticides damage our nervous system, impairing both mental and physical functioning, and leading to neurodegenerative diseases like Parkinson's disease,[8] autism, multiple sclerosis and more. In Alzheimer's disease, where the brain proteins are misfolded, leading to what are called neurofibrillary tangles and beta-amyloid plaque in the brain, pesticides are implicated,[9] as are heavy metals.

The other major types of pesticide, the carbamates and the neonicotinoids, are similarly neurotoxic (damage the nervous system – ours as well as that of the bees) and carcinogenic (cancer-causing). Pesticides are strongly implicated in many types of cancer,[10] especially cancer of the breast,[11] prostate and colon; all extremely common these days. The herbicide glyphosate, for example, has been seen to stimulate the growth of breast cancer cells in the laboratory, even at doses as low as parts per trillion. These substances damage the DNA in our chromosomes, and that's serious; it means that the damage will extend to future generations.[12] Glyphosate therefore leads not only to cancer but also to fertility problems, miscarriages, premature births and birth defects.[13] The younger you are, the more vulnerable you are to these toxic effects, so the foetus and baby are the most vulnerable of all.

Fertility in general and sperm counts in particular are falling right across the Western world, and pesticides are one of the major causes; organic farmers, who avoid toxic pesticides completely, have higher sperm counts than other men.[14]

Glyphosate has been categorised by IARC (International Agency for Research on Cancer, part of the WHO) as a probable carcinogen,[15] and its manufacturer, Bayer/Monsanto, has paid out over $10 billion to settle lawsuits brought by people who contracted cancer from contact with glyphosate. The first such claimant, Dewayne Johnson, developed non-Hodgkin lymphoma, a blood cancer, at the age of forty-two; he had been working as a school groundskeeper in California and had sprayed vast amounts of Roundup (one of the weedkillers that contain glyphosate) on the school grounds over the course of his career. I wonder how many of the school children got sick, too? And if so, did anyone make the connection?

One particularly scary thing that the glyphosate molecule does is to wrap itself around an atom of aluminium and take it right through the blood–brain barrier, into the brain. Aluminium in the brain is a very bad idea, as we'll see in chapter 2 on heavy metals. It is strongly associated with the development of Alzheimer's disease and has also been linked to autism. Some formulations with glyphosate in them already contain other toxic metals such as arsenic, lead and nickel, massively increasing their cytotoxicity (being directly toxic to our cells; 'cyto' is from the Greek word for cell). So, unless we are eating organic, we're getting a mixture of pesticides AND toxic metals: not a happy combo. And formulations like Roundup, which contain glyphosate together with other substances, turn out to be even more toxic to our genes than glyphosate alone.[16]

In my clinical practice, I have seen numerous cases of pesticide poisoning, rarely recognised as such by the medical establishment, but clear as day by taking a careful history and doing the right tests. Usually the poisoning is chronic (cumulative low-dose exposure over many years) as in Melanie's Story on page 30. But sometimes it is acute (a large exposure all at once) and sometimes it can be both. Acute pesticide poisoning remains a huge problem globally; in one year alone, China had 48,000 such poisonings, including 3,000 deaths.[17] And that's just those that got reported as such. Among those who suffer acute pesticide poisoning and survive, a proportion will go on to develop cancer or another serious disease in the years that follow; none of these illnesses will be recorded as deaths caused by pesticides.

As if it weren't enough to be neurotoxic and carcinogenic, these pesticides are also EDCs – endocrine disrupting compounds. This means they mess with our hormones,[18] including thyroid hormones[19] and the sex hormones oestrogen and testosterone. They are strongly implicated in our epidemics of premenstrual syndrome, obesity, thyroid disorders and type 2 diabetes, as well as in cardiovascular disease. Many of them act as oestrogen mimics, sitting on the oestrogen receptors on cell surfaces and interfering with the signals our cells are sending to each other; this is another way in which they are implicated in breast cancer, which is getting commoner every year.

Prostate cancer is also a hormonal cancer and turns out to be excessively frequent among men who work as pesticide applicators.[20] I see posters everywhere each November, inviting men to grow a moustache to raise awareness of prostate cancer. The ads say: 'Whatever you grow will save a bro.' Raising awareness is good, of course, as is expressing solidarity. But eating organic – not eating carcinogenic, endocrine-disrupting pesticides – might save an awful lot more bros than growing a moustache.

The glyphosate molecule, as its name suggests, is very similar in its chemical structure to glycine, an amino acid (constituent of protein), which serves many essential functions in the body. One of these functions is the synthesis of collagen, the main structural protein of our connective tissue, such as tendons, ligaments and so on. If glyphosate displaces glycine in our connective tissue, which is entirely possible, that's going to weaken our musculoskeletal system quite considerably. There certainly do seem to be a lot of musculoskeletal problems around, keeping the rheumatologists and orthopaedic surgeons very busy. Indeed, if glyphosate displaces glycine in ANY protein, that protein is going to look 'wrong' to the immune system cells, which may then start to destroy it. There you have the beginnings of autoimmune disease: the body in self-destruct mode. Examples of autoimmune diseases of the connective tissue and musculoskeletal system include rheumatoid arthritis, systemic sclerosis and systemic lupus erythematosus (SLE or lupus).

Glyphosate is causing kidney failure in young agricultural workers in Nicaragua and El Salvador,[21] who spray it on the sugar cane and absorb it through ingestion and inhalation and the skin; they don't have protective gear. In the twenty years up to 2016, it is estimated that twenty thousand people have died from this disease, known euphemistically as 'chronic kidney disease of unknown origin' (CKDu), in central America. And a comparable illness is rife in the rice paddy fields in Sri Lanka. According to the latest research, however, it's not of unknown origin: it's glyphosate poisoning. Glyphosate causes liver damage as well; for more info on this, do consult Dr Stephanie Seneff's disturbing but important book, *Toxic Legacy*.[22]

Glyphosate and/or similar pesticides are in our daily bread unless we buy organic bread or make our own from organic flour. They are in our fruit and veg, again unless it's organic. However, we don't only encounter pesticides in our food. They're in our tap water unless we filter it. They're on the grass in the park unless our local council has stopped spraying, as more and more mercifully have, thanks to the campaigns of the Pesticide Action Network UK. They're in the air if you live on or near a farm where pesticides are being sprayed; there is no legal obligation for the farmer to warn the neighbours when spraying is going to happen, and locals do get ill.[23] More and more scientists are calling for them to be restricted or banned.[24]

We can inhale these poisons as well as eating and drinking them, and people who work with them can also absorb them through the skin. Golf courses are the most heavily sprayed green spaces of all, a problem that is worse in the US than in Europe.[25] I wonder if anyone has done a study into cancer rates among golfers and the caddies who carry their kit? A recent study of a herbicide commonly used in the US (called 2,4-D) showed that people really have got this stuff in their bodies and that children are most at risk.[26]

Our pets are exposed too, from flea collars and direct application of flea-killing insecticides to their fur (safe, alternative ways to prevent pet fleas are described in Fleas on page 176), and even from rolling on the grass in the park or on roadside grass verges if those have been sprayed. One vet told me recently that he'd noticed cancer becoming much commoner in dogs than it was twenty years ago, and that dogs are not living as long as they used to.

The pesticides that are killing us humans and our pets are also lethal for wildlife; bees and butterflies, frogs and toads and birds are suffering and dying as well.[27] If you know any of the good people who work for conservation charities like the RSPB, do tell them this. Pesticides are a major reason for the drastic decline in the numbers of wild birds and thousands of other species of animals and plants. We share most of our genes and biochemical pathways with them, after all.

Herbicides like glyphosate (technically an organophosphonate, not an organophosphate, but the same kind of toxicity, or worse) not only kill the vital bacteria in the soil, they do the same to the vital bacteria in our own intestines.[28] In other words, over time, they mess with our gut microbiome, leading to digestive disorders and thus also, eventually, to many of the diseases of modern civilisation. Health (or illness) begins in the gut. And what happens in the gut, begins in the soil.

The manufacturers of glyphosate, Bayer/Monsanto, have claimed that it is harmless (I kid you not) for the following reason: it works by blocking a metabolic pathway (a series of vital biochemical reactions) that occurs in plants and bacteria but not in human cells. Technically, this is true. But here's the catch: this pathway (known in biochemistry circles as the shikimate pathway) does occur in the beneficial bacteria who inhabit our own digestive tract. And those friendly gut bugs are not just friendly, they're essential; increasingly, they are considered to be an organ of the body in their own right. They make many vital nutrients for us like B vitamins, biotin, vitamin K and butyric acid that we can't make for ourselves, they liaise constantly with our immune system and they have a big impact on brain function too. When glyphosate kills them, we get ill; it's as simple as that.

Furthermore, the way glyphosate (Roundup) works in the field is by preventing plants from taking up essential minerals from the soil. So, any crops grown with it are not only poisoned, they are also nutritionally depleted. This is a major reason why so many of my patients, eating an apparently healthy diet full of fruit and veg, turn out on blood testing to be startlingly deficient in the very minerals and vitamins that those foods should contain (and did contain, seventy years ago). This leads to fatigue and to countless other symptoms, which are described in the Farm without Synthetic Fertilisers section on page 23, because many mineral deficiencies can result from the use of synthetic fertilisers, as well as from glyphosate. Organically grown food, by contrast, is not only free from pesticides and synthetic fertilisers; it's also richer in essential nutrients.

Despite all this, extraordinarily, you can still buy Roundup and similar glyphosate formulations, for garden use, in any hardware shop or supermarket in the UK. I'd suggest that you don't. However, you could go in and ask the manager why they're still stocking this lethal stuff. The more of us ask, the sooner they'll stop selling it.

Of course, all this damage that glyphosate does is aimed at killing 'weeds' in the fields – but how come it doesn't also destroy the food crops themselves?

The answer is: genetic engineering. The crops grown with glyphosate are 'Roundup ready' – genetically modified to be able to withstand it. This doesn't make them healthy or safe, it just means they don't die in the fields like the other plants around them do. The use of pesticides is inextricably linked with the use of genetic engineering, which is why the big chemical companies who produce pesticides are buying up seed companies, hand over fist. Big Chem is in control of much of global agriculture now. But organic farmers are fighting back hard, and so can we as consumers. Regenerative and organic farmers can manage without pesticide use because they prevent pest infestations naturally, by encouraging natural predators and by maximising diversity.

2. Maximise Diversity

In nature, you always find a great variety of plant and animal species cohabiting. This way they all thrive. Nature doesn't make monocultures. Monocultures – massive fields of just one crop, which sadly we see all over the English countryside these days – are an open invitation to whichever pesky pests like to feast on that particular plant to go forth and multiply and eat it all up. The conventional farmer responds or prevents this by zapping the whole field with toxic pesticides. And then when the pest becomes resistant, the farmer adds another pesticide – and another. This is what I'd call an 'intervention cascade' – one artificial input leading to the need for another. (I've borrowed the term from women's critiques of obstetric practice. It applies to most of drug-based medicine too.)

But regenerative farmers don't need to get into that toxic vicious circle. They are mirroring nature by growing lots of different plants together. The resultant complexity means that any potential pests and weeds face a lot of competition. Gardeners call this 'companion planting'; garlic and marigolds, for example, can prevent unfriendly bugs from colonising the neighbouring plants.

I'm surprised to discover that this diversity extends to growing more than one crop together in the same field at the same time, and just separating them after harvest. At Gothelney Hall in Somerset, farmer Fred Price also gives me a warm welcome and a tour of his multi-generational family farm. He shows me a field with not one, not two but three crops growing all together: oats, barley and peas. They help each other, he explains, as each crop takes different nutrients from the soil, and each hosts different soil microbes. It's a win-win. He calls it inter-cropping or poly-cropping.

Among the three crops I can see some other plants, too, at low levels. Some farmers would call them weeds, but Fred explains that they actually do no harm, and don't get out of hand because the density, diversity and careful rotation of the main crop plants suppresses the 'weeds' just fine. Fred never uses herbicides; he wants, he says, to grow crops that are safe for everyone to eat. There is a bakery right there on the farm, milling his wheat into flour, and making it into safe, wholesome bread that you can give to your children without fear of glyphosate poisoning.

Fred says that he learns something new every season, by listening to the land. Farmers like him are not on automatic pilot: they are receptive to nature, seeing what works well and continually adapting to nature's own ways, rather than trying to force nature to accommodate to any preconceived ideas. Fighting against nature never works: it's a lose-lose.

Fred also has some very healthy pigs, who live outdoors all summer. The pigs help to fertilise the arable fields in between plantings. And, unlike factory-farmed pigs, they almost never get ill. If one did, Fred would call the vet, but he has very seldom had to, and he has never given routine antibiotics. (More below about the dangers to us from agricultural antibiotics.) Fred does his bit for wildlife, too, without losing any food-growing capacity. There's a corner of the farm, 10 per cent of his land, he says, which is constantly flooding (there are a lot of floods in Somerset). It can't be used for growing food, so he has let it develop naturally into a wetland habitat. Win-win.

3. Use Cover Crops

In between rotations of the main 'cash' crop, regenerative farmers plant 'cover crops', which are legumes that fix vital nitrogen into the soil. Because it's 'fixed' by these clever plants, it doesn't leach out into the groundwater whenever it rains. (In contrast, synthetic fertilisers do leach out, causing appalling damage downstream, about which more later.) As well as providing a natural source of renewable nitrogen, the cover crops do several other things:

They cover the ground, protecting it from the excesses of sun, wind and rain. Bare earth, I've learned, is a bad idea, and almost never occurs in nature. The earth needs its 'duvet of living plants' (a term coined by farmer Rebecca Hosking, of whom more below), which produce atmospheric moisture through transpiration (releasing water from their leaves). They capture sunlight and turn it into food, and their roots feed all the vital microscopic creatures under the ground. They hold nutrients in the soil, and just by being there they suppress weeds. And of course, they capture carbon from the atmosphere and return it to the earth. All this is in addition to the fact that as the plants die they turn into on-the-spot compost, as in your garden.

Yet if you drive around our green and pleasant land, you see that much of it is in fact a brown and unpleasant land – there's bare earth everywhere. Bare soil can't hold water (no plant roots to take the water up) so rain runs off it, contributing, paradoxically, to both floods and drought. Cover crops provide 'green manure' or 'living mulch', a source of organic matter that not only improves the soil's fertility, but also prevents it from eroding and blowing away, which is what happened in the 1930s Dust Bowl disaster in America (where the soil literally blew away in massive clouds of dead, dry dust). It's still happening – it's called desertification – but regenerative farming can reverse it and is doing so in many parts of the world. In fact, on regenerative farms, the layer of topsoil actually becomes deeper, not shallower, over time, thus becoming more fertile and progressively better able to produce food and sequester carbon, providing a major solution to world hunger and climate change. It's right there, under our feet.

4. Conserve the Soil Structure

This is 'no-till' agriculture. Ploughing apparently destroys the long filaments (hyphae) of the crucial soil fungi and ruins the delicate network of tiny air pockets that the earthworms and other creatures have been busy making. It's also not good for the earthworms themselves. (The earthworm count on Pipers Farm has been going up year on year, Peter tells me. That's a real sign of soil health.) Ploughing also releases carbon dioxide into the atmosphere; untilled soil can hold more carbon and it holds water better, too. Lastly, ploughing literally turns the ecosystem that is the soil upside down. This means, Peter explained to me, that the anaerobic microbes who live underground end up on the surface, exposed to oxygen and sunlight, which they're not evolved to cope with. Conversely, the surface creatures, who *need* oxygen and sunlight, find themselves buried underground, which is not their natural habitat, without either. So, many soil-dwelling creatures that help plant growth and nutrition are bound to die, every time the soil is ploughed.

I was completely astonished to discover all this; haven't farmers been ploughing, one way or another, for thousands of years? Yes, they have, says farmer John Cherry, founder of the Groundswell Conference on Regenerative Agriculture, but that's why soil fertility has been progressively declining and farmers' yields have gradually decreased. Apparently, this has been a problem going back to the earliest civilisations. From the Romans turning the bread-basket that was North Africa into the Sahara desert that we know today (and it's still expanding) to the 1930s Dust Bowl of the American Midwest, overexploitation of the soil is as old as agriculture.[29] But it's got much worse in the past century; as John Cherry points out, ploughing with horses or oxen would disturb the top few inches of the soil only, but modern tractors disturb it down to a much deeper level.

A word of caution here. No-till agriculture is an excellent thing, but on its own it's not enough. We also need to be certain that our food is truly organic – uncontaminated by pesticides and grown without synthetic fertilisers. I believe that some farmers who have adopted the no-till method to conserve their soil are still using herbicides (weedkillers) – if you want to be sure, enquire and explore!

5. Agroforestry

We are used to thinking of farms and forests as separate entities. But trees can and do form part of the landscape of farms. They do all the good things that all green plants do, but more so. And they're perennial. So, on regenerative farms, you can see trees coming back to the arable land – this is agroforestry – and indeed you can see animals grazing not just on grass but on the leaves of trees; this is called silvopasture, from the Latin *silva*, meaning a forest. Peter Greig says that when he trims his hedgerows, if he sees an oak tree sapling growing in the hedge, he leaves it well alone.

Despite what we're told by the agrichemical corporations who control the lifeless arable mega-farms, we don't need to choose between growing food for humans and conserving wildlife. Regenerative farms that are producing good food for the health of our bodies simultaneously provide a haven for the wildlife that's essential for the health of our souls, as well as for its own sake.

6. Farm without Synthetic Fertilisers

Regenerative farmers maintain soil fertility with natural organic matter, from plant compost as described earlier and from animal manure as I describe later. So, they don't need synthetic fertilisers. By contrast, in a field whose soil has been eroded and rendered subfertile by decades of ploughing and intensive overfarming, the farmer may feel the 'need' to use synthetic fertiliser. There's a vicious circle here, because synthetic fertilisers are a dangerous short-term fix; over the longer term they actually *decrease* soil fertility, as well as increasing soil erosion.

Initially, these fertilisers lead to a growth spurt but, because they contain only one or two of the nutrients that plants need (whereas natural compost provides the whole lot), the result is imbalance: fast-growing but spindly plants that do not provide the nutrition that humans and other animals require. Some such soils need to be rescued by the application of mineral supplements, much like many of my patients. I can't help noticing how similar this chemical farming approach is to that of modern medicine: give a synthetic drug that may help for a bit, but in the long term does harm, partly by being toxic in itself but also by neglecting the patient's needs for multiple nutrients. Industrial medicine and industrial agriculture have a lot in common: tunnel vision in the appliance of science.

To be nutritious for us, plants need lots of different minerals, not just nitrogen, phosphorus and potassium, which is all they get from synthetic fertilisers. I've never found a patient to be deficient in nitrogen, phosphorus or potassium. But I'm constantly finding people deficient in magnesium, zinc, selenium, iodine, chromium (III) and manganese. That's largely because these nutrients are all missing from the soil when it's not regeneratively farmed. These mineral deficiencies have numerous effects on our health:

- Magnesium deficiency makes it hard for muscles to relax, for the brain to work properly, for the heart to pump normally, for us to sleep properly and for the mitochondria (the energy-producing organelles in our cells) to work well and produce enough energy for us.
- Zinc deficiency affects taste and smell and stops the immune system doing its job of fighting off infections. In young children, zinc deficiency can stunt growth quite seriously. And we always find both zinc and magnesium deficient in children with autism and ADHD.
- Selenium is also vital for the immune system and is involved in preventing both infections and cancer.
- Iodine is essential for the thyroid gland and for the health of the breast, ovary, prostate and other organs; I always find it terribly low in women with breast cancer.
- Chromium (III) and manganese are essential for blood sugar control and assorted enzyme reactions in the body, as are magnesium and zinc too.

All these deficiencies and the ensuing illness and exhaustion can result directly from overuse of synthetic fertilisers and failure to replenish the soil's true fertility, but they can also result directly from the use of the herbicide glyphosate. Glyphosate prevents plants from taking up even such minerals as do remain in the soil, so it gives us a 'double whammy' of deficiency + poison. In the form of Roundup, it's the most widely used pesticide of all. If it's in the soil in which your food was grown, it's in your food. Avoid it – eat organic.

The synthetic fertilisers, by the way, were developed from explosives, and they do occasionally explode, as happened in Beirut in August 2020, with the loss of hundreds of lives. And that wasn't the first time. Their history, like that of the pesticides, is rooted in warfare. The chemical companies just repurposed them when the war was over. It's important, I think, to know where these things came from.

In *We Want Real Food*, and quoted with his permission, Graham Harvey describes precisely how the use of synthetic, chemical fertilisers for intensive farming is damaging human health.

> High output comes at a cost. In nature there's a phenomenon known as the dilution effect. While you can stimulate a crop to produce more per acre, the total nutrients produced are more or less fixed. All you get is more grains containing fewer trace elements or vitamins. In the same way a cow can be goaded into producing higher yields, but the resulting milk will contain fewer health-promoting vitamins per litre. The principal result of chemically-driven agriculture is dumbed-down food. Nitrate fertilisers promote ill-health. They weaken plants by stimulating excess growth of sappy tissue with thin cell walls. Crops grown this way are more prone to disease, which is why they need constant spraying with pesticides to keep them standing. And when fed to livestock, they make animals sick. Hence the need for routine antibiotics. It should come as no surprise that they contribute to human illness too.[30]

That is a very clear example of the intervention cascade in action.

The nitrates from synthetic fertilisers often end up in our water supply and have been associated with all sorts of illnesses including cancer of the colon and rectum, thyroid disease and neural tube defects like spina bifida.[31]

Synthetic fertilisers do another type of damage too. Combined with bare earth and excess tilling, their effect is to render the soil so fragile that it literally washes away in the rain. The soil, along with its content of nitrate and phosphate fertilisers, ends up flowing down rivers into lakes and the ocean. What the fertilisers do there is to make those waters as fertile as hell – they cause a bloom of blue-green algae.[32] These are not technically algae; they're phytoplankton, now known as cyanobacteria. They cover the water in a thick film, which uses up all the oxygen that's dissolved in the water. Fish die, whole aquatic ecosystems are destroyed. The result is vast dead zones (the official term is eutrophication, but 'dead zones' says it better).[33] Ironically, the waters have been rendered sterile by fertilisers, by an excess of nutrients. The worst example globally is the huge dead zone in the Gulf of Mexico, due to run-off of synthetic fertilisers from the industrialised agriculture in the Mississippi River basin.[34]

In the UK, the water companies spend a fortune trying to remove the nitrate fertilisers and pesticide residues from our water supply. They don't succeed very well at all, but still they pass on the cost to us as consumers. So, we pay, as opposed to the polluter paying. Something's very wrong here. Government action could turn this around – but we need to pressure them to do it. Maybe we should refuse to pay our water bills until the agrichemical industry is forced to clean up its own mess?

7. Integrate Animals, Naturally Pastured

What cows and other animals eat, and how they live, has great significance for human health. If cows eat primarily grass, which is what their stomachs have evolved to digest, their meat or milk will be rich in the healthy omega-6 fatty acid CLA (conjugated linoleic acid), which lowers our risk of cancer, heart disease, diabetes and obesity. It will also be rich in omega-3 fatty acids, which are vital for healthy brain development, in essential minerals like iron and zinc and in vitamins A, B and E. If the cows are fed on grain, however, or soya, they end up with a higher fat-to-protein ratio, and also a higher sugar load, so are more likely to be contaminated with pathogenic bacteria, which love sugar. Yet all over the US, farmers are growing soya and wheat and corn to feed not people, but cows. Why? Because they get massive government subsidies to do so.

In much of the UK, where there used to be grass and wildflower meadows, grazed by animals, we see instead vast empty fields of wheat that goes to feed captive animals (who would be healthier out on the grass) and to power the junk food industry (making us ill and vastly increasing the burden on the NHS) or to be burnt as 'biofuels'. And we see vast fluorescent yellow fields of oilseed rape. Rapeseed has been grown for centuries but its oil was used for lamps and candles, not food. Now it's allegedly been rendered fit for human consumption, but it's all genetically modified, and most of it is highly processed, hydrogenated, full of trans fats and has been 'cleaned' with the toxic solvent hexane. When in flower it is greatly exacerbating the nation's hay fever. It is a very profitable crop – and totally unnecessary.

What is even more insane (but again, highly profitable for some) is that our precious rainforests are being cut down to grow soya to feed cows. At time of writing, ClientEarth, an environmental law charity, is taking the American food company Cargill to court for cutting down rainforests to grow soy to feed animals, which end up as meat in our supermarkets. Not only do we desperately need the rainforests, which are the lungs of planet Earth and the richest ecosystems in the world, home to indigenous peoples as well as countless flora and fauna, but cows shouldn't even be eating soya. Or grain. They should be eating grass.

However, 'grass' turns out to be an oversimplification. The best regenerative farmers actually feed their cattle on 'herbal leys': pastures containing many species of legumes and wild herbs as well as grass. The cows, whether beef or dairy cattle, prefer this, and it makes them even healthier than grass alone. The herbs include many that occur naturally in wildflower meadows, such as yarrow, burnet, chicory, plantain, vetch, clover, sorrel, knapweed and dandelion. (Many of these herbs have medicinal uses in humans; they're good for us as well as the cows!) Cows who can eat these plants freely make more of the beneficial CLA than those who have only eaten grass. Grass on its own, with no other plants, I've learned, is another artificial monoculture.

In nature, plants and animals live together. Animals on farms fertilise the soil, returning both carbon and nutrients to the earth, eliminating the need for artificial fertilisers. They can regenerate the soil just as the aurochs, the wild ancestors of cows, did. Those ancient ruminants roamed around freely; however, they didn't stick in one place the whole time. Now regenerative farmers are mimicking nature in this respect too, finding that both the plants and animals are healthier if the animals graze one small patch intensively for a day and are then moved on, not returning to that patch for several weeks or months. It's often called 'mob grazing'. The grass gets the benefit of intensive grazing, the land then has plenty of time to recover and the animals get to eat tall, full-grown grass, including the nutritious seed heads and fibre, whereas, as one farmer delicately put it, 'young grass just goes straight through them'.

Peter Greig describes how his mob grazing works: the cows – who do look very healthy and contented in their wildflower meadows – only eat about one third of the grass before they are moved on. Another third they trample into the earth, so it acts as mulch (surface compost; the worms will take it down below) and one third remains growing in the field. The third that remains growing in the field Peter describes, using a term coined by Rebecca Hosking, as 'a green solar panel'; in other words, there is still enough green cover there to absorb sunlight and convert it into energy, which is what grass does. It's what all plants do.

Mob grazing is a version of holistic planned grazing, a method originally created by Allan Savory in Zimbabwe, and pioneered in the UK by Rebecca Hosking. On her organic, regenerative farm in South Devon, Rebecca moves her sheep to a different pasture every day, walking the fields and taking into account the ecology of what she sees growing in each patch. She notes rare species of wildflowers or birds, for example, and ensures that the sheep don't graze where skylarks are nesting or orchids are growing; the sheep will come back to those areas when the flowers have set seed or when the birds have finished raising their young. This is love of nature in action.

Grazing animals kept in this manner not only provide healthy meat, milk and wool, they actually help to reverse both soil erosion and climate change. The concern about cows contributing to global warming by belching methane only applies significantly to the vast industrial factory farms called CAFOs (concentrated animal feeding operations, or 'feedlots'). In these ghastly places, hundreds of thousands of animals are kept squashed together in extremely inhumane conditions, frequently get ill, and produce not only excess methane but also so much concentrated 'manure' that it can contribute, like synthetic fertilisers, to the dead zones described previously. The animals in these nightmare factory farms are the ones eating the soya for which the rainforests are being destroyed. A circle of complete insanity.

These CAFOs began in the US but sadly exist in the UK too now, where they are known as 'mega-farms'. I am not a vegetarian, but I would never eat meat from such a place. Furthermore, animals kept in cruel and crowded conditions and fed on food they weren't evolved to eat are bound to have lowered immunity. To prevent the infections that would otherwise be rife, the farmers give them routine antibiotics. Intensively reared pigs and chickens, as well as some beef cattle, are fed on regular low-dose antibiotic drugs that then get peed out, ultimately, onto the earth. There they damage the soil bacteria and find their way into the water table and into us humans. And if we eat the meat of these animals, we are ingesting the antibiotics directly. In tiny doses, yes, but regularly, and the cumulative effect is significant.

Peter Greig describes how, in his past as an intensive chicken farmer, he was supposed to stop all antibiotic treatment five days before the chickens were slaughtered, so there would be no antibiotics left in their systems. However, he said, the middlemen who came to collect the chickens were sometimes in such a hurry (due to pressure of demand from the supermarkets, and/or others in the absurdly long supply chain) that he was instructed to cut corners. The chickens were picked up on a Thursday, not the following Monday as required by law, and still had the antibiotics in their systems.

What do these regular, low-dose antibiotics do to us when we eat such meat? First of all, they kill some of the essential, friendly bacteria in our gut – the microbiome (or, as I call it in *SAITT*, our Trillions of Tiny Companions). Second, partly as a direct result of that, they weaken our immune system. Thirdly, it is possible that antibiotics damage our mitochondria, the energy-producing organelles in our cells. This is likely because evolutionary biologists think that our mitochondria were originally bacteria, living symbiotically inside our cells. They certainly do resemble them under the microscope. So, a drug that damages bacteria may well damage our mitochondria. The main symptom would be fatigue, and there's a lot of that about. The highest density of mitochondria occurs in brain cells and muscle cells; hence, mental and physical fatigue.

Even more worryingly, this drip-drip of unintentional antibiotic intake leads inevitably to resistance; the evolution of bacteria that can't be killed by antibiotics. The routine administration of antibiotics to farm animals, in addition to the too-frequent medical prescribing of antibiotics, puts all of us at risk. It means not only that our gut microbiome gets damaged, and the immune system along with it, but also that antibiotics, which should be used sparingly, may not work in the emergency situations where they really are needed. Eating only organic, regeneratively farmed meat can avoid these risks to a very great extent.

I've learned from Peter's, Fred's and Rebecca's farms that herbivores allowed to live a free and natural life don't need antibiotics and can contribute hugely to fertilising the soil, reversing desertification and feeding/clothing us humans well and safely. Thank goodness for regenerative farmers like them, who have shown that you can farm well (and make a living) without toxic chemicals and without cruelty. These farmers have turned from vicious circles to virtuous cycles. They are not just refraining from doing harm; they are actively rebuilding the soil's structure and fertility, giving us humans a last chance to eat real food and to survive and thrive on this amazing blue-green planet. If many other farmers can be enabled to follow their lead, we will hopefully have far more than the fifty or sixty harvests that – the UN predicted – remain to us.

As I leave the farms, I find I'm thinking about one of my patients. I'll call her Melanie.

MELANIE'S STORY

Melanie grew up on a very different kind of farm. It was a large arable farm in a flat part of the UK, growing wheat and other cereals. Her dad sprayed his crops regularly with chemical pesticides. There were no animals grazing on the farm, so no animal manure, and Melanie's dad didn't rotate the crops or apply organic matter (compost) to the soil. He used frequent applications of synthetic nitrate fertilisers. Melanie has a vague early childhood memory of seeing birds around the farm but says that by her teens they had mostly disappeared.

Melanie says that she and her sister played around the farm after school and were never told to go inside and close the windows when the pesticide spraying happened. She does, however, remember that one of her father's employees who was involved in the spraying was diagnosed with Parkinson's disease at the early age of forty-three. There is an established link between pesticides and Parkinson's disease.[35]

Melanie herself came to see me with a different problem. She had breast cancer. She was forty-seven and had two teenage children. The oncologist she had seen wanted to do chemotherapy first, to shrink the tumour, and only then refer her for surgery. He said that the surgery would be less extensive that way, 'giving a better cosmetic result'. Melanie was dubious about this; she instinctively felt more anxious about chemotherapy than surgery, and wanted the tumour removed ASAP, before she proceeded to any other treatment. So, after a considerable struggle with the 'system', she had managed to have the operation before she came to see me, and, unlike most cancer patients who have consulted me, she had not been through chemo or radiotherapy.

Melanie was, of course, desperately upset about her diagnosis, and was asking herself the inevitable question, 'Why me?' In my practice of ecological medicine, I take this question seriously; I do not regard it as rhetorical or just an emotional reaction. It is, in fact, the key question doctors should be asking themselves about every illness in every patient: 'Why has this happened?' In Melanie's case I was looking for all the possible contributing factors, in terms of nutritional deficiencies and environmental toxins, because if we can find causes we are a long way towards safe, effective treatment, as well as prevention of recurrence.

In taking a detailed history from Melanie, I learned the facts described above about her childhood on the (not remotely organic) farm. The first thing to do, then, was to test her, not only for nutritional deficiencies but also for the presence of pesticides. Most organophosphate (OP) pesticides are 'lipophilic'; this means they dissolve in fat, not water, so they are unlikely to be found by a blood test unless the exposure was yesterday – the body quickly hides such toxins away in the fatty tissue. So, I took a fat biopsy. (Fat is liquid in the body, so this is just like doing a blood test but with a wider needle, usually taken from the thigh or buttock. Sadly, it is very hard to get this type of test in the UK now.)

Melanie's results showed the presence of not one but three different pesticides. I found high levels of glyphosate, the main ingredient of the common weedkiller Roundup, even though it is actually water-soluble. And I found moderate levels of two other organophosphate pesticides: tetrachlorvinphos and parathion. The organophosphate pesticides were derived originally from nerve gases used in the two World Wars, therefore, unsurprisingly, are often toxic to the brain and nervous system. But they can also damage the endocrine (hormone) system, the reproductive system, the gut microbiome (vital friendly bugs in our digestive tract) and more. They can also cause cancer; the International Agency for Research on Cancer (IARC) classifies glyphosate as 'probably carcinogenic to humans' and it classifies tetrachlorvinphos and parathion as 'possible human carcinogens'. These two have, in fact, been banned in the EU and UK. But they were not banned when Melanie was growing up on the frequently sprayed farm.

Melanie was astonished when I shared the test results with her. 'But I haven't lived on the farm for twenty-nine years!' she exclaimed. 'How can they possibly still be in my system?' A genetic test provided the answer to this mystery: Melanie had a glitch (the technical term is a 'polymorphism') in the gene that makes the enzyme paraoxonase 1 (PON1), which is capable, to some extent, of detoxifying the organophosphate pesticides. So, she couldn't break down and excrete the pesticides very well. This glitch is very common and may explain why so many people are made ill by these common toxins, while others, at least for a while, are not. Furthermore, Melanie's exposure to these toxic chemicals had occurred during her childhood; children, even those without this genetic glitch, produce less of the PON1 enzyme than adults do.[36] (This is one of many reasons why the young are the most vulnerable to these toxic exposures.)

There was another mystery to be solved. Melanie confirmed with her father (still alive although not well) that he had used Roundup (which contains glyphosate) on his crops ('Everyone did; everyone does,' he said) but he had no recollection of using the other two chemicals. Parathion used to be used on vegetables, and there was a small vegetable garden by the farmhouse, so he might have used it there. 'He certainly sprayed something on the veg, to keep the weeds down, but none of us looked at the ingredients list,' Melanie said. And what about the tetrachlorvinphos? That's an insecticide used on animals; Melanie's dad didn't have cows or sheep on his farm. However, she recalled, they had dogs and cats at home, and her mum or dad would periodically put 'something' on them to kill fleas. That would fit.

Of course, I cannot conclusively 'prove' that the pesticides Melanie encountered in her childhood and that we found in her body were the same molecules exactly, or that they were the cause of her breast cancer. Plenty of people develop cancer without having had that kind of childhood, and other people who live on agrichemical monocrop farms do not get cancer (although a disproportionate number do[37]). And all of us encounter these kinds of chemicals all the time, in repeated low doses, if we eat non-organic food. But then, one in two of us now get cancer, which wasn't the case a hundred years ago, and our food crops are drenched in these toxic chemicals, which also wasn't the case a hundred years ago.

Either way, it made no sense to leave carcinogenic pesticides in the body of a person with cancer so, with Melanie's consent, we embarked upon a detoxification programme. I won't describe this in detail, as detox methods are covered in *SAITT* on pages 297–307. But suffice it to say that Melanie had a challenging regimen, which included daily organic vegetable juicing, twice-weekly saunas, high-dose vitamin C and other supplements such as vitamin D, glutathione, PC (phosphatidyl choline), omega-3 and omega-6 fatty acids, iodine and a little selenium.

I also asked her to cut out sugar completely (it feeds cancer cells), and to eat only organically grown food and nothing processed, so she was consuming no synthetic additives, just real food. I ensured she ate nothing that came in a plastic package, and didn't use plastic water bottles or plastic wrap, because plasticiser chemicals contribute to breast cancer too; they are as bad for us as they are for the oceans – more on this in chapter 3. Furthermore, I encouraged Melanie to eat plenty of the foods that are thought to be protective against breast cancer: grapefruit, raspberries and the brassica vegetables (broccoli, cabbage, cauliflower, kale, watercress and Brussels sprouts).

The importance of eating organic for someone like Melanie (for all of us, in fact) cannot be overemphasised. Otherwise, she would be consuming daily doses of pesticides like glyphosate, which had made her ill in the first place. These doses would be tiny but cumulative, and would defeat the object of the detox, as she would be doing a minuscule 're-tox' with every meal.

Within weeks, Melanie felt great on this admittedly demanding programme, and she also noticed that her immune system was strengthened; she used to get coughs and colds all the time, she said, and those stopped, while her energy level improved. Both a strong immune system and good energy production are crucial for preventing cancer from recurring, or from occurring in the first place. A year after her initial visit we re-tested; the pesticide residues were gone.

Melanie decided, after a lot of thought, not to go ahead with the chemotherapy that the oncologist was urging her to have. This wasn't just fear of the dreadful side effects. She had done some research and had also read *Curing the Incurable* by Dr Jerry Thompson,[38] an experienced GP. She had discovered that although chemotherapy initially shrinks tumours, it only prolongs life in 5 per cent of cancers, and most of those are blood cancers such as leukaemia. Some studies, she found, have shown that chemotherapy actually increases the incidence of metastases (cancer spreading)[39] and others have shown that, in breast cancer and similar cancers, chemotherapy increases survival rates by barely over 2 per cent.[40] It seems, Melanie concluded, that oncologists use chemo because they have little else in their toolkit; other studies suggest, however, that they are quite reluctant to use it on themselves.

Melanie chose to say 'no' to radiotherapy too. Nine years later, she is very well and remains cancer free. A postscript to her story concerns her sister, Caroline. I had asked quite early on whether Caroline, who grew up in the same conditions, was alright. Melanie said that she was 'OK-ish, but morbidly obese.' Caroline was intrigued by Melanie's decision and her drug-free recovery, so she came to see me and asked to be similarly tested for the presence of agricultural pesticides. I found all the same chemicals in Caroline's fat biopsy, at similar levels.

Caroline's experience was that every attempt to lose her excess weight had made her feel ill and exhausted, so she had given up. This makes sense; when you burn fat, any toxic chemicals stored in that fat will be released into the bloodstream and make you feel lousy. I explained to Caroline that, for this reason, detox had to precede weight loss. She considered it, but in the end decided against; it's a very demanding process.

There are numerous studies showing that today's obesity epidemic is linked with exposure to pesticides.[41] But why did the pesticides lead to breast cancer in one sister, and obesity in the other? Indeed, why do they lead to neurological disease like Parkinson's disease or dementia in some people, lymphoma in others, gut problems in others, infertility and birth defects in yet others? Everyone's biochemistry is different, and all of us are exposed to a whole cocktail of toxic chemicals, so it is rarely going to be possible to establish simple linear links between chemical A and disease B. Except for some occupational exposures, it is much more complex than that. But the overall picture is clear. We are poisoning ourselves, and we don't have to.

What Is to Be Done?
Questions, Actions and Resources

At this point, you may well be asking yourself the following rather obvious questions:

- If regenerative farming is so good for the soil and therefore for us, and if there is so much evidence that industrial farming is damaging our soil, our food, our health and our climate, then why on earth – pardon the pun – aren't *all* farmers changing over to regenerative / organic methods?
- If pesticides are implicated as contributory causes in the majority of modern diseases, why aren't they banned?
- If synthetic fertilisers erode the soil, produce toxic wastes and dead zones and are the major agricultural source of greenhouse gases, why are they still manufactured by the tonne?

These are good questions. In this section I will endeavour to provide some answers, and then suggest what we might do as individuals, as well as swiftly surveying the vast and encouraging range of collective initiatives that already exist and are campaigning for change with not-inconsiderable success.

First of all, we have to talk about politics. About power, money and greed. There is no escaping it. The huge chemical corporations who make the pesticides and synthetic fertilisers, the gargantuan junk food industry that processes food till it isn't even food anymore and all the middlemen in the 'food supply chain' standing between us and the farmers who ultimately feed us – they want their profits, all their profits and nothing but their profits. They don't want regenerative/organic farming because it stands in the way of those profits. They can't see past their profits to the bigger picture, to the earth as a whole, to the bleak, arid and hungry future that awaits even their own grandchildren if we don't turn food and farming around.

The classic response of those who care, when social change is urgently needed, has been to Speak Truth to Power. That may be noble and necessary, but I'm not sure it's sufficient now; I'm not sure power even recognises the language of truth. Power does, however, recognise the language of money. That's how we can get through to them. We can boycott their toxic goods, their junk food, their pesticide-infested lettuce and their cruelty-infested meat. We can find more and more ways to eat in such a way that their contaminated products become redundant, we ourselves become healthier and they either have to turn to truly regenerative methods or go out of business. As William Lana of Greenfibres says: 'What we buy will be produced, what we don't won't.'[42] These companies are big and powerful, yes, but they are ultimately completely dependent on customers. That's us.

We need to vote with our wallets. We can begin by finding ways to cut out the middleman, by buying our food more directly. There are more and more regenerative farms that sell directly to the public at the farm gate, but even in cities now there are increasing opportunities. You could start with the website of the Real Food Campaign, www.realfoodcampaign.org.uk. Then there's www.farm2fork.co.uk, which offers fruit and veg boxes from small, local producers. Some people imagine that they can't choose what's in their fruit and veg box, but most companies do enable you to choose your items online, rather than get a standard box.

If you eat meat, you could check out www.pastureforlife.org, whose meat is from animals exclusively fed on grass. Their certification ensures that the cows are 100 per cent grass-fed; they haven't been just let out in the fields for a bit, and then fattened up on grain indoors afterwards (there's a lot of that about).

Of course, we want to minimise imports, to reduce air miles. But as Graham Harvey points out, far worse environmental damage, including CO_2 emissions, is caused by lorries transporting food within Britain than by air freighting. He quotes studies showing that if we could all buy our food within 20 kilometres of where we live, environmental damage would be reduced by 90 per cent.[43] To find food that's grown locally you might also try www.findlocalproduce.co.uk or www.bigbarn.co.uk, though I haven't been able to ascertain whether they're always organic as well as local.

Another useful website is www.ooooby.com (that's the letter 'o' four times, not four zeros) – it helps you find a local organic veg box wherever you live, and there's minimal packaging, no plastic and minimal miles. In Scotland, www.locavore.scot arranges deliveries of locally produced fruit and veg. They also have Locavore shops in Glasgow, Edinburgh and other towns. A 'locavore' is someone who is trying to eat locally grown food.

Beware greenwashing in all its forms. Planet Tracker (https://planet-tracker.org) examines examples of greenwashing and helps you look out for it, and you can find more information in the Resources section.

'Now this is all very well,' I hear you say, 'but lots of people simply can't afford to do what you're suggesting. Never mind voting with their wallets – they're going to food banks just to survive!'

This is true. Outrageously, in one of the richest nations on earth, millions of people are living in poverty. This is what hypercapitalism (a term I first heard from Colin Tudge) does, and there is no excuse for it; it is just plain wicked. And what do people donate to food banks? Tins and packets. As Henry Dimbleby said (on a panel discussion at the British Library on 24 April 2023), 'We have one of the most unequal societies in Europe. But cheap junk food is not the solution to poverty.' Indeed, why should those who are poor be poisoned as well as poor?

The forces of greed that are keeping so many people desperately poor are the same forces that are destroying our soil and trying to feed all of us on junk. We are seeing unbridled selfishness in the economic sphere, with the rich growing richer and the poor growing poorer, hungrier and more poisoned by the day.

Nevertheless, whoever can afford to vote with their wallet, I would say, needs to do so. It is the ethical imperative of this moment. And junk food, by the way, is not really cheap at all. That's an illusion. We all pay the hidden price in the form of tax-payer-funded (ineffectual) environmental clean-ups of the mess created by intensive food production, processing and transport, attempts to remove agricultural chemicals from our water supply, damaged soil, increased sickness and a collapsing NHS. If industrial farmers, food manufacturers and supermarkets had to clean up the mess themselves, I believe organic food would end up being cheaper than non-organic.

All food could also be made genuinely cheaper if it weren't for the middlemen in between us and the farmers, taking their cut. Whatever you pay in a supermarket, the farmer gets less than 10 per cent of that, sometimes as little as 1 per cent. If it's processed food, like burgers, the food processing companies get ten times more than the farmer does – and all they've done for us is turn real food into junk food! A 'food manufacturing industry' is a ludicrous concept anyway; if it's manufactured, it isn't food.

There are, thankfully, more and more excellent projects designed precisely to enable the poorest in our society to eat the decent food that everyone deserves, and enough of it. One excellent organisation is www.foodfoundation.org.uk, which is working to improve children's diets, increase vegetable intake and influence government policy in the right direction, among many other initiatives.

What is the UK government doing about food and farming? At time of writing, sadly, they are making things worse; their farm subsidy system is just plain crazy. They give 80 per cent of their subsidies to the biggest 20 per cent of farms, which are almost invariably among those doing industrial, chemical, soil-eroding farming, and growing genetically edited crops. The small mixed farms, encouraging biodiversity and soil health and producing safe food, get virtually nothing. This is one of the major reasons it is so hard for farmers to transition from industrial to regenerative/organic farming; the economics just don't work for them. This destructive government action comes on top of pressure from the food-processing companies and supermarkets to 'grow those chickens faster!', as Peter Greig put it. The farmers, the chickens and the consumers all suffer from this, but the profits of the food-processing companies grow as obscenely fast as the battery chickens do.

Furthermore, many farmers are advised by agronomists, 'crop doctors', who are often employed by, and/or on commission from, pesticide companies or companies closely connected with those industries. Their advice almost always involves recommending the application of chemicals, much as the advice of medical doctors most often includes prescribing chemical drugs. The power of the pesticide companies over farmers is comparable to the increasing power of the pharmaceutical industry over medicine, both human and veterinary medicine. (It is rumoured that pharmaceutical firms are now deeply involved in funding medical education. I wonder if pesticide companies are similarly involved in funding agricultural colleges? I have no idea; I'm just wondering aloud. Might be worth looking into.) But in both farming and medicine, anyway, there's a large and growing holistic movement fighting back, challenging our dependence on unnatural, toxic substances, and finding gentler, safer ways.

Why might governments be hindering rather than supporting the development of safe, organic, human-scale farming? I don't know. But being generous, and assuming that nobody in any government has any financial ties at all to the pesticide or fertiliser industries, or to the genetically modified seed companies, which are increasingly the same as the pesticide companies, perhaps they are simply under the mistaken impression that organic, regenerative methods can't produce enough food to feed the people? Perhaps they've been listening to these chemical agribusiness conglomerates, who argue loudly and repeatedly that we absolutely have to use pesticides, fertilisers and genetically modified (GM) crops in order to feed the world's population, projected to be ten billion by 2050?

Maybe these multi-billionaires are genuinely concerned to prevent famine, or maybe they are genuinely concerned to maintain their power and profits. Either way, however, the evidence is all to the contrary. Numerous studies show that, when compared to conventional farms, regenerative farms not only produce crops and livestock with higher nutrient density (more vitamins, minerals, phytonutrients and essential fatty acids),[44] they actually produce greater yields overall.[45] More food, not less. So, we don't have to sacrifice quantity for quality or vice versa; we can have both. This is not really surprising. After all, as Colin Tudge points out,[46] traditional farming (small, mixed, family farms, no combine harvesters) is what allowed the world's population to rise from 10 million, 10,000 years ago, to 2 billion by the late 1920s. A 200-fold increase, with no input from chemicals or GMOs (genetically modified organisms). It works; it has always fed the people. At least, it did until the advent of colonialism.

I believe that together we can turn things around. History is littered with examples of successful public campaigns that have made great changes against all the odds. To select a tiny sample at random: women won the vote, seat belt laws were passed, lead was taken out of petrol, gay marriage happened and we got a tax on plastic bags. Oh, and a worldwide consumer boycott contributed significantly to the downfall of apartheid in South Africa.

There are countless marvellous campaigns going on right now, but I have to single out a particularly brilliant organisation, Pesticide Action Network UK or PAN UK (www.pan-uk.org).

I was very lucky to be able to interview two of the hardworking people at PAN, Josie Cohen and Dr Stephanie Williamson; I can only convey here a fraction of what I learnt from them. On the grassroots level, PAN are leading a campaign for pesticide-free towns. At time of writing, thanks to their campaign, fifty towns in the UK have gone pesticide-free (stopped spraying their parks and grass verges, etc.) and another seventy or eighty are on their way. The aim is a nationwide ban, and I think they'll achieve it. On the national level, they are working hard to persuade those in government at DEFRA (the Department for Environment, Food and Rural Affairs) to establish targets for a reduction in pesticide usage and toxicity. They know how to lobby; they are totally determined and they are skilled at speaking truth to power in a way that gets things done. And for the ordinary householder, you can download from PAN 'A Guide to Gardening without Pesticides'.

On the retail level, PAN UK rank the top ten UK supermarkets on how well they're doing at reducing pesticide-related harms linked to their global supply chains. This is making a big difference; the supermarkets know they're being watched, assessed and rated. Check it out at www.pan-uk.org/supermarkets. Apparently, supermarkets do test their produce for pesticide residue levels – more than the government do – but thus far only the Co-op and Marks and Spencer have actually published the data. PAN are demanding that the other supermarkets do so. If you shop at supermarkets, make sure to ask the manager, as often as possible, what they are doing to reduce and eliminate pesticides in their products. They want our custom, so the more we do this the quicker they will make the changes.

On the international level, PAN (www.pan-international.org) are fighting against the use of pesticides in cotton. A huge 95 per cent of cotton is grown with pesticides, and the cotton farmers and especially their children can get very ill. PAN's 2021 survey in India found that 47 per cent of cotton farmers reported poisoning in the previous year, and 12 per cent of these episodes were severe.[47] More info at www.pan-uk.org/cotton-poisoning. Overall, PAN UK tell me, 44 per cent of farmers experience pesticide poisoning.[48] African farmers are spending up to 60 per cent of their income on pesticides! That's great news for the pesticide manufacturers, but they don't pay the resulting healthcare costs. PAN have long-term projects in Benin and Ethiopia, working with the local people to grow cotton organically; it is perfectly possible. To make a difference to this, as well as for the sake of your own health, look out for 100 per cent organic cotton clothing (more about how to find this in chapter 3).

Paraquat is a very toxic herbicide now banned in the UK and Europe but, PAN told me, there is a factory still making it in Huddersfield in Yorkshire; they export it to countries where it's not banned. The same happened with DDT and the other organochlorine insecticides. In 1962, with the publication of Rachel Carson's epic *Silent Spring*,[49] the dangers of these persistent, polluting pesticides were revealed to the world. Rachel Carson was persecuted and vilified by the pesticide industry but, nevertheless, by 1972 DDT was banned in the US, and then other Western countries followed suit. Here's the catch; they were banned in the West but exported to Africa and India. This is a pattern.

Furthermore, much of what is being grown in the Global South are cash crops for Western consumption, rather than food for local consumption. People in Africa could feed themselves quite well – climate change notwithstanding – if they could simply grow what they need to eat, as they did before the White Man invaded. As far as I can see, economic colonialism continues unabated.

PAN have also co-founded The Pesticide Collaboration, which brings together health and environmental organisations, academics, trade unions, farming networks and consumer groups, working towards a shared vision to urgently reduce pesticide-related harms in the UK. There are more studies every year linking pesticide use to serious diseases such as cancer and Parkinson's disease; for a database that collects this information, see the American website www.beyondpesticides.org. And, of course, the Soil Association, (www.soilassociation.org) has been doing much fantastic work in the UK for many decades, including ensuring that any food that bears their logo really is wholly organic and, in the case of animal products, genuinely free range. We'll meet the Soil Association again in chapter 7.

CHAPTER TWO

EARTH II: HEAVY METALS

What we do to the earth, we do to ourselves.

Ted Perry, *Home*

Beyond the farms are the mines. For millennia, we humans have been digging metals out of the earth. Sometimes this is ok and sometimes it isn't; some metals – mostly 'heavy' metals – are toxic. Or rather, they're harmless when left in the earth's crust, but not harmless when dug up, and the processes involved in releasing them from their subterranean slumber and extracting them from their ores create serious pollution. Most of them are used industrially, and those who mine them or work with them are most at risk.[1] But all of us are affected to some degree. These heavy metals get into the soil from mining, from other industrial processes and from air pollution – the results of burning fossil fuels (see chapter 4).

Here are the main culprits; I've put their chemical symbols in brackets: aluminium (Al), arsenic (As), cadmium (Cd), chromium (VI) (Cr(VI)), lead (Pb), mercury (Hg) and nickel (Ni) are the most important toxic metals, and the ones I most commonly find in the body when testing sick patients. I and my colleagues in the British Society for Ecological Medicine have learnt how to remove these safely from the body; more on this later.

Less well-known but also potentially dangerous are antimony (Sb), barium (Ba), beryllium (Be), bismuth (Bi), gadolinium (Gd), palladium (Pa), polonium (Po), silver (Ag), technetium (Tc), thallium (Tl), thorium (Th), tin (Sn), titanium (Ti) and uranium (U). A longer but far more entertaining list can be heard by listening to the great Tom Lehrer singing his song 'The Elements': all one hundred plus elements of the periodic table – by no means all toxic! – sung to a Gilbert and Sullivan tune. (Check out the 1967 version from a concert in Copenhagen. I know, I'm showing my age.)

Metals are examples of elements, the simplest substances in chemistry, meaning that, in contrast to compounds like pesticides, they can't be broken down into smaller units. They're not made of other substances. An atom of silver, for example, is an atom in the original sense of the Greek *atomos*: that which cannot be split. (Nuclear fission notwithstanding, if you split an atom it ceases to be itself. It is no longer an atom of that metal or of anything else. It has lost its chemical identity.) Whereas a molecule (such as a protein or a pesticide) is compounded of several types of atom: it's made up of different elements.

This has big implications for what toxic metals do to our bodies if they get in. We cannot break them down. Our white blood cells, the sturdy soldiers of the immune system, can engulf them, but they can't dissolve them. It's as if they swallow them but cannot digest them. So, they carry them around, unwittingly facilitating their transport to all parts of the body and, most significantly, into the brain.

Toxic metals can cross the blood–brain barrier, and they all damage the brain; like pesticides, they are neurotoxins. They distort protein structures, leading to the neurofibrillary tangles and beta-amyloid plaque found in the brains of people with Alzheimer's disease. Indeed, autopsies have found high levels of toxic metals such as mercury and aluminium in the brains of people who died with dementia, autism, MS and other neurological conditions.

Nutritional Defences

In the body generally, much of the harm that toxic metals do is done by displacing the good metals, the vital nutrient minerals such as zinc. Zinc is an essential cofactor (helper) for up to three hundred different enzymes in the human body. (An enzyme is a large, complex protein molecule whose job is to catalyse – kick-start – a particular biochemical reaction in the body). An atom of zinc sits at a specific site on each enzyme molecule to enable that enzyme to do its job. But toxic metals like mercury, cadmium, lead or nickel can take the place of zinc on any of these enzymes, especially if we are zinc deficient. If there are, say, ten atoms of mercury floating around and only one of zinc, mercury will 'win' a place on the enzyme – and proceed to interfere with its function in the body. If, however, there are ten atoms of mercury but one hundred of zinc in that corner of your internal milieu, then zinc will win, and mercury will be pushed out.

This, in a nutshell, is why good nutrition is the single most important way to protect ourselves from toxic metals. The more of the good stuff we have inside us, the harder it is for the bad stuff to get a foothold.

All the toxic metals lead to neurological problems such as lower IQ, poor memory, behavioural disturbances and psychiatric illness. Equally, the majority of these metals are endocrine disruptors, mostly metallo-oestrogens; they sit on oestrogen receptors on cell surfaces and either suppress or amplify the 'oestrogen signal'. This can contribute to premenstrual syndrome (PMS), polycystic ovary syndrome (PCOS), fertility problems (male and female), delayed or accelerated puberty (depending on whether the oestrogen signal is suppressed or amplified), prostate problems and more. The thyroid and adrenal glands can get damaged too.

The toxic metals are also carcinogenic and there is a particularly strong link between aluminium and breast cancer. The toxic metals are among the substances implicated in our epidemics of autoimmune disease, such as rheumatoid arthritis (RA), multiple sclerosis (MS) and Hashimoto's disease, because they distort the structure of our proteins, fooling our immune system into seeing them as 'alien' proteins and attacking them.[2] The tissue that gets attacked is the joints in the case of RA, the myelin sheath around the nerve cells in MS and the thyroid gland in the case of Hashimoto's disease, which is autoimmune thyroiditis. Toxic metals also lead to kidney disease, liver disease – I could go on.

Is this all beginning to sound a little bit familiar? Yes indeed. It is almost identical to the list of problems that pesticides can cause! The corresponding good news, though, is that, if you do what you need to do to avoid pesticide exposure (eat organic, filter your water), you are simultaneously avoiding the majority of your potential exposure to toxic metals. Organic farms don't tend to be located on old industrial sites, but to be sure I wrote to the Soil Association to check that their regulations prohibit heavy metal contamination as well as pesticides and synthetic fertilisers. Here is their reply.

> Organic farmers are required to evaluate and manage any risk of contamination to your organic products by any unauthorised or prohibited substances and ensure measures are in place to reduce the risk of contamination. This includes heavy metals. If there are reasons to

> suspect that there is contamination of soils by heavy metals this will need to be tested for and managed. Any composts and some fertilisers that can be used in organic farming have to demonstrate that they don't exceed thresholds for heavy metal contamination.[3]

In an imperfect universe, that's as good as it gets, and it'll do for me.

At the end of this chapter, I'll take you through the environmental sources of the worst offenders in the toxic metal arena – because it's not only soil/food – and thereby show you how to minimise your exposure to them. I'll also explain briefly how you can find out 'what's got into you' and begin safely to remove these toxic metals from your system. But first, let's look at a real-life example of heavy metal poisoning and how I dealt with it. This is about mercury (Hg) and what it did to a little boy whom I'll call Finn.

FINN'S STORY

Finn is a young man now, but he was four years old when his parents first brought him to see me back in 2008 (the date is important; we'll see why shortly). He ran around the consulting room looking frantic. He knocked my stethoscope off the desk and then ran to the window, flapping his arms wildly, to watch the passing cars. Each time a car passed he yelled 'car' very loudly and flapped even harder. He wouldn't make eye contact with me or with his mum or dad, and he wouldn't leave the window. Between Finn's shouting, his parents eventually managed to tell me his story.

He had developed fine till the age of about fifteen months. He'd laughed a lot, crawled and walked at the usual times, babbled breezily at everyone, made eye contact willingly and was very happy to be cuddled. He had begun to say a few words. Around fifteen months, Finn had started to have screaming fits, pulling up his legs as if he had colic. He sometimes got diarrhoea, other times was constipated; his gut wasn't right. He began banging his head on the floor, which was most alarming, and he had begun to arch his back and go stiff in his parents' arms when they held him. He became very fussy about food, having previously eaten a wide range of suitably mashed-up foods, and refused all vegetables except, later on, pickled cucumbers, for which he was regularly raiding the fridge by the time I saw him.

He seemed to lose some of the baby words he had learned and his playing developed a rigid, mechanical character. He would line up his toy cars obsessively and would play with nothing else, and he stopped interacting with other children at the playgroup. He always seemed anxious and on edge, and occasionally had rather terrifying tantrums, far more extreme than the usual toddler tantrums.

By age four, Finn had a diagnosis of autism and was heading for 'special school'. His parents were desperate for him to go to an ordinary school and not be excluded, as they put it, 'from society at large'. They had been told, however, that Finn was quite severely autistic, and that was that. They had also been told 'it must be genetic', although they had scoured their respective family trees and found no relatives, living or dead, with anything remotely resembling Finn's neurological symptoms.

To make a difference, I needed to know what was going on with Finn's biochemistry. Blood tests were out of the question, but we did, with some difficulty, manage to obtain samples of hair, urine, stool and sweat. What showed up, as well as low levels of zinc and magnesium, was a moderate level of mercury in the urine, a high level of mercury in the hair and a very high level of mercury in the stool. Mercury did not appear in the sweat; some people are more vulnerable to mercury poisoning precisely because they cannot excrete it via sweat.

Mercury does not belong in the human body at all and is well known to be a neurotoxin;[4] it damages the brain. (The 'mad' Hatter in *Alice's Adventures in Wonderland* was not invented by Lewis Carroll; hatters used mercury in their work and were known to go mad.) The symptoms of mercury poisoning (and, to some extent, of poisoning by any toxic metal) bear a remarkable resemblance to the symptoms of autism. Once in the body, most heavy metals head for the brain, where they become incorporated into protein structure, altering the functioning of the neurones (nerve cells). Mercury also pushes healthy minerals, such as zinc and magnesium, out of the body, so was quite likely to be responsible for Finn's nutritional deficiencies. I also knew, from seeing countless other similar children, most of whom I *had* been able to blood test eventually, that Finn would have low levels of the B vitamins.

I had to work out a programme to begin to detox the mercury out of Finn's body. Giving supplements of zinc and magnesium and the B vitamins would be a good start, but only a start. I also wanted to know: Where had all that mercury come from? How had it got into him?

I took a detailed medical history from Finn's mum about her own health. She had been well all her life and remained perfectly well during her pregnancy with Finn. His birth had been natural and of normal duration, so brain injury from oxygen deprivation during labour (commoner than we think) was not the issue here. Digging deeper, however, I discovered that she had had poor teeth in her own childhood and had been given a number of metal amalgam fillings. These contain about 50 per cent mercury. Most dentists believe that the mercury remains in the filling and does not leach out into the rest of the body, but a vast amount of evidence now shows this to be mere wishful thinking.[5]

Finn was the first child in his family, and mercury from his mum's dental fillings would have leached out into her own bloodstream and from there through the umbilical cord and placenta into Finn while he was in the womb. This would have effectively 'detoxed' the mercury from his mum's body (she felt 'marvellous' throughout the pregnancy) but would have landed Finn with a problem: mercury poisoning.

It turned out that Finn also had another possible source of mercury in his system. He had had several early childhood vaccinations around 2005, the time when the UK and US authorities were removing mercury (in the form of thimerosal) as a preservative from vaccines (but adding in aluminium, also a neurotoxic metal, as an 'immune adjuvant'). At the time of the changeover, older batches of diphtheria and tetanus jabs still contained mercury. Of course, Finn's mum didn't know exactly what was in the vaccines he had had; how many parents ask to read the ingredients list in the manufacturers' package insert? Or indeed the list of potential side effects that's also in there?

Finn's mum decided, for her own sake and to protect future children she hoped to have, to get all her metal amalgam fillings safely removed, by a specialist dentist who stuck to the protocols of the British Society for Mercury Free Dentistry or the IAOMT, the International Academy of Oral Medicine and Toxicology. Dentists who belong to these societies know how to remove and replace the fillings without releasing mercury into the system, which is what would happen with the standard dental drilling method. Many people remove these fillings for symptom relief,[6] but in this case it was preventive medicine, reducing the risk of neurological disease in the future.[7]

We figured out that Finn got his initial dose of mercury through the placenta and seemed to tolerate that amount, but that subsequent doses in the childhood vaccines raised his body's total load to more than he could cope with; his liver's detox systems were overwhelmed and he manifested all the symptoms of mercury poisoning, or full-blown autism. (Other heavy metals, notably aluminium, can have similar effects, as Professor Christopher Exley has demonstrated; see below.)

Finn's parents confirmed that he'd seemed alright after the first set of immunisations, was irritable after his second batch, agitated and unwell after the third lot and developed a high fever with non-stop screaming and crying after the fourth set. They had taken Finn to A&E on this occasion and had been reassured that, although it had gone on for many hours, it was 'a natural reaction' and not to worry; it would pass. Nevertheless, it was from this point on that Finn gradually, between twelve and fifteen months, began head-banging, withdrawing from social contact and having screaming fits.

Detoxifying mercury out of the body is possible but challenging, especially in a young child. It was always going to be a slow process. As well as the three supplements mentioned above, I gave Finn vitamin C, chlorella, coriander, selenium, iodine and PC (phosphatidyl choline). The vitamin C was powder dissolved in orange juice, as was the chlorella, but that had to wait till he was six years old. Finn's parents just integrated fresh coriander leaf into as many meals as possible. Coriander, like chlorella, is brilliant at picking up mercury and removing it from the body, BUT it is equally good at picking up mercury from industrially contaminated soil. So, we had to ensure that all the coriander Finn consumed was organically grown. The zinc (in liquid form) toned up Finn's taste buds, so he became less of a fussy eater (though he remained obsessed with pickled cucumber) and that widened the range of foods he would eat. This in turn enabled us to introduce into his diet the sulphur-containing foods: onions, garlic and leeks. Sulphur is an element that also helps to detoxify mercury out of the body. So, we had a virtuous cycle.

Selenium and iodine also help to remove mercury and we gave them in very tiny doses in liquid form from time to time. PC is a liquid best consumed by children when mixed into yogurt with berries, and Finn was very happy to eat this. Another important substance that helps the body to detoxify heavy metals is glutathione, but we had to wait till Finn was ten and could swallow capsules before adding this to his regimen. Interestingly, a genetic test we did at this stage (a saliva test; he still couldn't tolerate a blood test and there was no need to put him through it) showed that Finn's body was not very well able to synthesise his own glutathione, so his detox capacity would always be slightly impaired. This 'glitch', like Melanie's lack of the enzyme PON1 (see Melanie's Story, page 32), which can detox OP pesticides, is very common in the population.

Along the way, as well as heroically getting all these supplements into Finn, his parents chose, with my support, to follow the dietary protocol pioneered by Paul Shattock OBE of Sunderland University. This involves omitting all foods containing casein (dairy protein) and gluten; for many autistic children on this plan, eye contact improves, social contact improves and gut problems and other symptoms begin to resolve too. The proposed mechanism is that the proteins gluten and casein, when incompletely broken down, are absorbed as neuroactive peptides into the bloodstream and have an opioid-like effect. Although formal studies have shown variable results,[8] in Finn's case (and that of many others), we saw significant improvement within four months of starting this programme. He became more relaxed with physical contact with his parents, could look people in the eye, and his playing became more natural, less fixated on cars. His screaming fits stopped altogether.

Finn didn't end up in a special school. His parents home educated him until he was six, by which time he was considered well enough to be admitted into mainstream school. As he grew into his teens, further detox modalities became possible for him, such as saunas and organic vegetable juicing and the herbal remedy milk thistle, which helps the liver with its detox tasks. Epsom salts baths have been helping Finn since I first saw him; that's how we got the magnesium into him. Epsom salts are magnesium sulphate. The magnesium calms both mind and muscles, and the sulphate assists some of the liver's detox pathways.

When Finn reached eighteen, I wanted him to have a few sessions of colonic hydrotherapy for extra detox, but he has drawn the line at that. He is nineteen at time of writing, at university and functioning far better than anyone expected. Like many autistic people, he is excellent at maths and physics. He is still autistic, and would rather spend his evening with a maths problem than at a party, but he can form friendships and has had his first girlfriend.

His gut function has improved significantly (for how to do this, see 'Spring Cleaning your Gut' in chapter 2 of *SAITT*), so he can digest proteins properly, including some gluten and casein, so he no longer needs to be on the restrictive diet that helped him so much in the early days.

I re-tested Finn every two years till age eighteen, and we saw his mercury levels slowly going down. At the last two re-testings, age sixteen and eighteen, the level had, finally, reached zero.

There are two more pieces of good news connected with Finn's story. His mum, having had all her mercury amalgam fillings safely removed as described above, and having then followed a detox programme herself for a few months to remove any residual mercury from her system, conceived another child, a boy, and three years later a little girl. Both children are completely well, with no signs of autism. Not only have they received no mercury via the placenta, they have also not been vaccinated. Childhood vaccines in the UK no longer contain mercury, but many do contain aluminium, which is also a neurotoxin, and Finn's parents just didn't want to take the risk. Finn's siblings are well protected from infectious childhood diseases by having been breastfed, by eating well and by getting plenty of sunshine, fresh air and exercise.

The second piece of good news concerns legislation around mercury. A total ban on mercury in dental fillings is on its way. The UK is somewhat behind most European countries on this; Sweden and Norway announced a ban in 2008 and other countries are following on. The UN Minamata Convention calls for a total phasing out of mercury in all its uses. The EU is banning the use of dental amalgam from 1 January 2025. In England, Scotland and Wales, mercury fillings are now, finally, illegal (with some exemptions) for children under fifteen and for pregnant or breastfeeding women. The British Dental Association is resisting these changes at every step, insisting that mercury may be a problem for the environment, endangering wildlife and so on, but poses no risk to human health. This is sadly illogical; we humans share most of our genes and most of our biological processes with wildlife. If it damages plants and animals, it damages us.

And, God bless the NHS, here's what their website said about this in May 2023: 'There is no evidence that exposure to mercury from amalgam fillings has any harmful effects on health.' There are several thousand academic published papers that they clearly haven't read.[9] Funny, though, that they have phased out mercury-containing thermometers and sphygmomanometers (blood pressure measuring devices) on grounds of toxic risk – but they think it's still ok to put the stuff into our mouths!

And now, let's spare a thought for the people who handle this dangerous liquid metal and inhale its vapours as part of their occupation. This includes dentists and dental nurses,[10] of course, who have more than their share of neurological disorders, but I'm thinking here of the impoverished workers in Mexico, China and other places who mine it, extracting it from its ore, cinnabar. Sounds like cinnamon, I know (same reddish colour – it used to be used to make the red pigment vermilion) but not nearly so pleasant. It is mercury sulphide (HgS) and extracting the mercury from it is associated with neurological illness, disability and death among both cinnabar miners and some gold miners.[11]

Why gold miners? Here's why: about one fifth of the world's supply of gold comes from illegal 'pick and shovel' operations in Asia, Africa and South America, the small-scale, unregulated gold mines. The miners use mercury; they combine it with the gold to make a solid amalgam, which they then heat, to separate out the gold. They inhale the mercury vapour, with all its associated health risks,[12] and the process also releases mercury into local waterways, degrading the environment.[13] (I only learned this recently; I've been wearing a gold ring for several decades, but I couldn't trace its origins. Can you trace the origins of any gold jewellery you might be wearing? The supply chains of gold are no more transparent or traceable than the supply chains of junk food.)

The Minamata Convention aims to change all this. As one (mercury-free) dentist who attended the convention in 2022 told me,[14] dentists who still use mercury amalgams are reselling the spare mercury back to the unregulated gold miners – and so it goes around. Let's just hope that, as this particular vicious circle is broken by international legislation, efforts are also being made to find other, safer employment for those miners.

Toxic Metals: The Seven Main Culprits and a Few Minor Ones

For each of the seven major toxic metals, I'll tell you its environmental sources (and therefore how to avoid it), what it does to the body and how to get rid of it from your system. But I should warn you, if this gets a bit repetitive, it's because the sources of most of these poisonous metals are very similar, and the effects of many of them in the body and brain are similar, as well as what to do about them, although there are a few important differences.

All of them are released by mining and smelting, and almost all of them are released again by the burning of fossil fuels. This is because they exist, in small amounts, deep in the earth, so the coal etc. that we dig up and burn contains some of them. Let's stop right there and take in the implications of that for a moment; we're all worrying about the climate effects of fossil-fuel burning, and rightly so, but there are also other, I would say equally compelling, reasons why we need to massively reduce the burning of coal and oil and gas. Apart from the various toxic gases released, nanoparticles of toxic metals are released too, and we're inhaling them on our streets. More on this in chapter 4.

In terms of symptoms, the majority of these metals do most of the damage described above, just before Finn's story, but there are also certain problems particular to certain metals. I'm primarily concerned with the effects of long-term, low-level exposure, the invisible drip-drip of daily contact with them and the chronic diseases that result. But if you look them up, you'll mostly see the effects of a one-off accidental exposure to a large amount ('acute' as opposed to 'chronic' exposure, and quite rare).

In regard to treatment and/or removal, there are certain nutrients that help remove almost all of these toxic metals, such as vitamin C, the B vitamins and zinc, but again there are certain nutrients that are especially good at removing certain particular metals. So, let's get into the specifics:

Arsenic (As)

Arsenic is a metal, and a toxic one at that. It is used as a pesticide in its own right and as a component of other pesticides, particularly for (non-organic) rice. Mostly this is in countries where these things are not well regulated, but if we are eating food imported from those countries we are at risk. Similarly, in some countries it is not illegal to use arsenic in animal feed. It gives chickens 'leaky gut' and makes them absorb all their food faster, so they grow fatter quicker,[15] giving a shorter time to slaughter: more profitable. Arsenic also makes chicken meat pinker and 'more attractive to the consumer'. Adding it to chicken feed for these reasons is perfectly legal in the US, but not in the EU. And in the UK? At time of writing, the legislation is still in a post-Brexit muddle.

Arsenic in drinking water is a particular risk if artificial fluoride (hexafluorosilicic acid) has been added to the water supply; hexafluorosilicic acid may be contaminated with arsenic and adds on average about 0.08 ppb (parts per billion) of arsenic to our tap water. Invest in a water filter! (See chapter 3 for more information.) Arsenic has also been found in cosmetics, American baby food, American protein powders and protein drinks, spray-on tanning lotions and in triple super phosphate (TSP). This last is a common fertiliser used in the UK – so if it's in the fertiliser, it's in the soil, it's in the food on your plate. Avoid it by eating organic!

Arsenic in the human body does much of the damage described above, including being an oestrogen mimic and increasing the risk of precocious (early) puberty and many cancers, among them cancers of the breast, prostate, colon, lung, liver, kidney, bladder and nasal passage. Arsenic can damage the brain, liver, kidney and lungs, and contribute to type 2 diabetes. It can cause raised blood pressure and abnormal heart rhythm, thickening and roughness of nails and skin, drowsiness, confusion, convulsions, muscle aches, pins and needles, numbness, anaemia, infertility, miscarriage, low birth-weight babies and neurodevelopmental disorders such as low IQ, cognitive impairment and learning disabilities.

Of course, all these symptoms and illnesses can have other causes as well; arsenic toxicity may or may not be a contributing cause in any particular case. So how do you know if arsenic is a problem for you? The simplest way to find out whether you are carrying this or any other toxic metal is to get tested – I can highly recommend Viva Health Laboratories (www.vivahealth labs.com) in the UK, Micro Ttrace Minerals lab in Europe (www.microtrace.de), or Great Plains Laboratory (www.mosaicdx.com) or Doctors' Data (www.doctorsdata.com) in the US. But you will need to be referred by a practitioner. There is a list of suitably qualified practitioners on my website (www.drjennygoodman.com) and a good practitioner won't just order the tests for you, they'll take a proper medical history. And ideally, you'll let them interpret the results for you and help you work out a treatment plan.

I have seen some patients with arsenic poisoning, though fewer than with the other toxic metals. In most cases we couldn't figure out the source, and in one case the patient actually suspected malfeasance! But standard detox protocols got rid of it within six months, and the symptoms – mostly neurological – improved substantially. The basis of the detox approach is in *SAITT* on pages 297–307, but it always involves high-dose vitamin C (building up the dose gradually to your personal maximum) and zinc, saunas, organic vegetable juicing and ensuring that all necessary nutrients, especially the minerals, are at optimum levels. One of the reasons that treatment really needs to be personalised is that your particular nutritional deficiencies may be contributing, and they can't always be guessed at; they may need to be tested for.

In terms of prevention, research shows that good defence against poisoning by arsenic is provided by a healthy microbiome. Probiotics, whether from supplements or fermented foods like kimchi, kombucha and kefir, reduce the absorption of arsenic from the gut into the bloodstream.[16] And the same is true for other heavy metals. Remember, antibiotics damage the gut microbiome and probiotics replenish it.

Nickel (Ni)

Nickel is found in stainless steel, which many cooking pots are made of, and it leaches out if you cook something acid in the pan, such as tomato or fruit. (See chapter 7 for info on safer pots and pans.) Body piercing is a concern too, as the metal used tends to be stainless steel; pure silver or gold are safer. Nickel is used in the manufacture of margarine; another reason to avoid margarine (a synthetic junk food that is bad for our cell membranes) like the plague! Organic butter is just fine. Nickel is used in some dental materials and heart stents and is in cigarette smoke and vapes. It is in some cosmetics, and in belts and buckles including the fastenings on bra straps; some people, particularly women, can develop a direct sensitivity to nickel, when any contact with it will trigger a rash or full-blown dermatitis (skin inflammation). Where there is nickel sensitivity there is usually nickel toxicity, so, if you find your skin reacting badly to contact with metal, nickel toxicity is likely.

Nickel is in car fumes, released by catalytic converters and also directly from the stainless steel in the exhaust pipes themselves. These nickel particles are so fine that our lungs cannot filter them out, so we can't cough them up; they go straight into the bloodstream. Nickel, like arsenic and other toxic metals, is also found in TSP fertiliser, so the advice above applies again. Don't eat it! Eat organic!

Nickel does the usual heavy-metal damage, including acting as a metallo-oestrogen, and is especially good at displacing zinc from vital enzymes. In particular, nickel is implicated in cancers of the breast, ovary and lung, in childhood leukaemia and in disorders of blood sugar control, both hypoglycaemia (low blood sugar) and diabetes. Nickel from urban traffic pollution has been linked to heart disease.

However, we have plenty of experience with getting rid of nickel successfully. It requires lots of zinc and vitamin C, but also an amino acid called methionine, which, in the presence of sufficient zinc, can 'chelate' nickel and carry it safely out of the body. The zinc displaces the nickel and the methionine grabs onto it and removes it. Ideally you would work with a practitioner to do this, but there is a good basic treatment protocol for nickel detox on Dr Sarah Myhill's website (www.drmyhill.co.uk – go to 'Toxic problems' and then to 'Nickel'). Dr Myhill recommends glutathione as well as methionine; this is a detox molecule that we are supposed to produce in our own bodies, but some of us do so better than others. Most people I see with toxicity issues produce less than the optimum amount of glutathione, so it makes sense to add that into the regimen. You can get a genetic test to find out how well your body makes glutathione from www.lifecodegx.com.

Chromium (VI) (Cr(VI))

I've put this one next because in practice I usually find it in the same patients in whom I find nickel. They have similar sources, including stainless steel exhaust pipes and dental appliances, cookware and clothing fasteners, cheap jewellery, cosmetics and, again, TSP fertiliser, which you won't be eating if you eat organic. Chromium (VI) is also used in leather tanning, wood preservatives and some dyes and is found in waste from steel and pulp mills and metal-plating industries, which can end up in our water supplies.

Chromium (VI), or chromium-6, is also known as hexavalent chromium. It is a toxic, carcinogenic, endocrine-disrupting metal. In contrast, chromium (III) (Cr(III)) – chromium-3 or trivalent chromium – which is the same element in a different chemical form, is not only harmless but actually necessary in tiny amounts for glucose metabolism.

Hexavalent chromium is the toxin that got into the groundwater in Hinkley, California, as a result of a gas pumping station operated by PG&E, the Pacific Gas & Electric company. People got sick: asthma, bronchitis, nosebleeds and assorted cancers. Animals got cancer too. This was all documented and exposed by the heroic campaigner Erin Brockovich, as you can see in the 2000 film of the same name. Of course, the company denied and dissembled for as long as possible before they paid up. The compensation, such as it was, can of course never compensate for lost lives and lost health. And it's not over; my understanding is that, despite the revelations, the 'compensation' and the fame of the film, the land and water are still contaminated and people are still sick.

There are similar towns, with different toxins contaminating them, all over America. There are some in the UK too; see Appendix II for more. One of the lessons here is to be alert to trends, to patterns of sickness; if you notice lots of people getting sick where you live, there is a reason. It may take courage, determination and a lot of detective work to find out what's going on. But it can be done.

I detox chromium (VI) with the same methods that work for nickel, and it seems to go away within six to nine months, based on re-testing results. Of course, as with any toxin, the thing is to try to identify the sources, to prevent 're-toxing'.

Cadmium (Cd)

This is a particularly nasty one and should be better known.[17] It's in tobacco smoke and, unlike the tar in your lungs or the nicotine in your bloodstream, it doesn't disappear over time when you give up smoking. It's produced by combustion of fossil fuels – car fumes again! – and other industrial processes, and it's in certain types of yellow paint. I once found it at extraordinarily high levels in an artist who was very sick indeed and used to paint with his fingers rather than a brush, using oil paints. It was going into him through his skin as well as his lungs. Cadmium is also released by the burning of rubber (tyres) and plastic, especially yellow plastic, and yet again it's in that toxic fertiliser TSP. It has been found in infant soy formula, American protein powders and drinks, and in sweets, cosmetics and hair products. It may be in battery acid, motor oil, brake linings and rubber carpet backing too.

Cadmium gets into the bones and causes bone disease, including severe bone pain. It's implicated in arthritis (both osteo- and rheumatoid) and osteoporosis; it displaces calcium and it inhibits the osteoblasts, the cells that make and remake bone. It interferes with the sense of smell (possibly by displacing zinc) and it's yet another metallo-oestrogen, linked with cancers of the breast,[18] ovary and womb. IARC (the International Agency for Research on Cancer) classified cadmium as a group 1 carcinogen back in 1993. It damages the heart, lungs, liver, kidneys, nervous system and pancreas, and is implicated in diabetes. Cadmium was found, along with lead and other toxic metals, in the urine of 'special' children in a children's centre in Punjab, an area of India that the West has long used as a dumping ground for its own toxic waste, including heavy metals and pesticides. These children had suffered neurological damage as a result.[19]

Detoxing cadmium is, frankly, difficult, but it can be done. As well as using the usual measures – an organic diet, water filter, tip-top nutrition (especially zinc, which cadmium displaces), high-dose vitamin C, saunas, organic vegetable juicing and so on – I have usually found it necessary to refer such patients to colleagues who can do intravenous detoxing. They may use vitamin C intravenously, and/or they may use other substances like PC (phosphatidyl choline) I/V to remove the cadmium. They describe cadmium as 'sticky' – it doesn't want to leave the body, so you have to persist.

A word of warning, though. You should only go to an experienced doctor for intravenous treatment, never to one of the high-street shops springing up around the place offering I/Vs as 'boosters' or 'detox' or whatnot to all and sundry. That's not personalised medicine. Putting anything into the bloodstream is a serious matter. And even with a doctor, they should take a detailed medical history for at least an hour, and they should work with diet and lifestyle measures with you for some weeks or months before proceeding to intravenous treatment. If they don't plan to do that, go somewhere else! (See list of recommended colleagues on my website). For most purposes, nutritional therapists, naturopaths and so on are every bit as good as doctors, and arguably better than most. But for intravenous treatment, no.

As with arsenic, the good news is that healthy bacteria in the digestive tract will reduce the absorption of cadmium and ensure that more of it is excreted in the faeces. If in doubt, take some probiotics and – especially if you've been unlucky enough to have to take a course of antibiotics – replace the good bugs that will have been slain by taking probiotics as soon as you've finished the course of antibiotics.

Lead (Pb)

The first thing to notice about lead is that its chemical symbol appears to bear no relation to its name. But the Latin for lead is *plumbum*, and that's where we get the word 'plumbing' from. Pipes carrying water were made of lead for hundreds of years, and some people suffered lead poisoning as a result. There is even a theory that lead poisoning contributed to the fall of the Roman empire; the Romans replaced their stone aqueducts with lead pipes, used lead for cooking utensils and for pots in which they pressed grapes to make wine (the acidity would have leached out the lead), and used lead to make plates, jewellery, cosmetics and more. Lead is a neurotoxin, so this could account for the bizarre behaviour of some of the later Roman emperors. Cognitive decline combined with falling fertility, both of which would result from high lead levels, could have done more damage than barbarian hordes to the Roman empire. We can never know for sure.

Unlike the other metals under discussion, the neurotoxicity of lead is very widely acknowledged. Lead used to be used in petrol as an 'anti-knock' agent, and numerous studies showed cognitive decline and neurodevelopmental disorders in children living near heavily polluted roads. The good news: lead was taken out of petrol some years ago in the Western world. The bad news: it was replaced with benzene, not a metal but a toxic compound, implicated in leukaemia. Sorry! (Another reason why we need fewer cars on the road, whether petrol or diesel. More in chapter 4.)

Lead is still found in the paintwork (and pipe work) in very old houses and most of the lead toxicity I have seen in the clinic has been in people who have been paint-stripping such houses to do them up. Lead is in some products imported from countries that have not banned its use: plastic toys and children's jewellery from China, cosmetics such as kohl used in Asia and the Middle East and also other cosmetics including spray-on tanning lotions, eye shadow, mascara, lipstick and hair dyes. As with the other toxic metals we've looked at, lead is released from the burning of fossil fuels, and found in that dreadful fertiliser TSP, and its entry into the body and brain is facilitated by fluoride.

Lead causes high blood pressure and other damage to the cardiovascular system, interferes with red blood cells, acts as a metallo-oestrogen to delay puberty in girls and mess with testosterone in boys, and can lead to infertility in both men and women. Most of all, it damages the brain and nervous system, leading to numerous disorders from deafness and blindness to memory loss, convulsions, muscle weakness, Parkinson's disease, motor neurone disease,[20] psychosis and more. It damages the foetus and leads to severe behavioural disorders in children exposed before or after birth.

Lead also damages the liver and kidneys and it heads for the bone. Once there it can lead to arthritis, cartilage destruction and osteoporosis, but it also represents a danger just by being there; during pregnancy and breastfeeding, and at menopause, lead may be released from the bones into the general circulation, and from there it can reach other organs including the brain. This means we have to be very careful about detoxifying lead; sometimes it is safer to just leave it in the bones than try to release it. Detoxing lead is a specialist area, and there are particular substances used to do this, although it is less and less needed in the Global North these days.

However, in the Global South it is another matter. In Zambia quite recently, children living near a lead mine were found to be seriously poisoned with lead.[21] Indeed, I have had an adult patient from Zambia who used to play around such a mine as a child and had very high lead levels on testing, even decades later. He had heart problems, blood disorders, neurological disease and more, and is one of the few people whom I was unable to make significantly better.

Preventively, again we find that probiotics help, by reducing the body's absorption of lead as well as other toxic metals.[22]

Aluminium (Al)

Aluminium is the most abundant metal and the third most abundant element in the earth's crust; only oxygen and silicon are more plentiful. So, there's a lot of it about and, for about 130 years, industrialists have been finding more and more uses for it. The problem is that aluminium has no role in the human body at all. It doesn't fit with our biochemistry and it would be better for us if it stayed where it belongs, under the ground.

Aluminium gets into us from aluminium foil if we wrap it around any acidic food (that could be meat or fish or vegetables on which we've squeezed lemon juice) or if we cook acidic food like fruit or tomatoes in an aluminium pan. (See chapter 7 for discussion on safer cookware.) Furthermore, aluminium is in some antacid drugs for indigestion, takeaway containers are often made from it and it's in some cosmetics (again!) and in antiperspirants and deodorants. These last are very important, as the aluminium goes into us through the skin of the armpit (and if it stops you sweating it stops you detoxing!) and is strongly implicated in breast cancer.[23] Most serious of all, however, is the aluminium that is being injected directly into us if we have the annual flu jab, and which is also in many babies' and children's vaccines, including the HPV jab that is offered to teenage girls; I have seen many of these girls get incredibly sick afterwards, for a distressingly long time.

Aluminium in the human brain is a contributory cause of Alzheimer's disease[24] – a major epidemic – and is strongly implicated also in our epidemics of autism and other neurodevelopmental disorders; it was mercury that poisoned Finn, but I have seen toddlers and older children with similar effects, more recently, from aluminium.

Ironically, given that aluminium is put into vaccines as an 'immune adjuvant' – to stimulate the immune system to react more strongly to the vaccine – it is the immune system that is frequently damaged by aluminium. Aluminium certainly does its job of making the immune system 'react more strongly' – but it seems to react indiscriminately, not in a targeted fashion, and I've seen people end up with autoimmune disease in just about any organ of the body.

How to get aluminium out of the body? As well as all the usual methods described above, there is one particular substance that, luckily for us, specifically pulls aluminium out of the body. That substance is naturally occurring silica, in its bioavailable form as silicic acid. Chemically, silicic acid is one atom of the element silicon surrounded by four hydroxyl groups, each composed of one hydrogen and one oxygen atom. It works. I and my colleagues in the BSEM have all seen aluminium levels fall and patients get a lot better using silica in this form to enable the body to excrete aluminium. Silicic acid grabs on to aluminium much as methionine grabs onto nickel and pulls it out of the body. It can take from six months to two years to get to zero, depending on the initial aluminium load (measured by Viva Health Labs or other labs as above) and on how intensively the person is able to put the detox regime into practice. And on how assiduously they avoid 're-toxing' with aluminium; the hardest thing is persuading people that they don't need deodorants. If we wash regularly and eat healthily, we really won't be smelly!

And just as with the other heavy metals, if you do ingest aluminium, a healthy microbiome will help you excrete much of it rather than absorb it into the bloodstream.[25]

To find out lots more about aluminium and what it's doing to us, check out Professor Christopher Exley's excellent book, *Imagine You Are an Aluminium Atom* (New York: Skyhorse Publishing). Professor Exley is a world expert; he has been studying the biochemistry of aluminium for about forty years. His preferred version of silicic acid to remove aluminium is that found in a naturally occurring mineral water from Malaysia, marketed as Acilis (silica backwards) in the UK. (There is some silica in Volvic water too, but not quite as much.) I was reluctant to use Acilis when it was only available in plastic bottles (see chapter 3 for why) but now it is available in glass bottles I would happily use it. However, I have tended to use the herb horsetail, which preferentially absorbs silica from the soil, and the supplement, Silicon Organique, from LLR G5, an originally French company based in Ireland. Any and all of these are good options.

Mercury (Hg)

We've already looked at mercury, but there are some environmental sources of it not mentioned in Finn's story. His mercury came from his mum's fillings and from the thimerosal preservative in his childhood vaccines in the early 2000s. But there are other important sources including, sadly, fish. Industrially produced mercury ends up in the ocean and pollutes the plankton, which get eaten by the little fish, which get eaten by the big fish – mercury gets concentrated at the top of the food chain. So big fish contain far more mercury than little fish. For this reason, in my view, it's ok to eat smaller fish like sardines and mackerel, but not big ones like tuna. And, as with almost all the other toxic metals we've mentioned, the burning of fossil fuels is a major source of mercury pollution; mercury levels in the biosphere are at least four times higher than they were in the 1880s.

As well as contributing to neurodevelopmental disorders like autism, ADHD and more, mercury is yet another metallo-oestrogen, and also interferes with the thyroid gland, is linked to stillbirths and cerebral palsy, gynaecological problems like endometriosis and PCOS and to adult neurological disorders like Parkinson's disease,[26] Alzheimer's disease, MS and motor neurone disease. It is strongly linked to heart disease including abnormal heart rhythms (arrhythmia), high blood pressure, tachycardia (fast heart rate), damaged blood vessels and cardiomyopathies (heart muscle damage). Mercury damages the gut microbiome; it used to be used as an antibiotic for syphilis and has the capacity to kill good bacteria, opening the field to an overgrowth of yeasts, unfriendly single-celled fungal organisms, in the digestive tract. It leads to autoimmune diseases and is implicated in chronic fatigue syndromes, fibromyalgia, eczema and more. But I'll stop there.

There are a few more toxic metals we must mention. Titanium (Ti) is used as a (totally unnecessary) white colouring in 'foods' such as milk powder, icing sugar, sweets, chewing gum and certain soy milks and also in toothpaste, sunscreens, cosmetics and the 'safety coatings' on low-dose aspirin. Shockingly, it's even in some nutritional supplements – the cheap and nasty ones. (See how to avoid them in chapter 6 of *SAITT*.) Animal studies have shown titanium causing the same kind of damage described above for most of the other toxic metals.[27] And the European Food Safety Authority (EFSA) declared in 2021 that titanium dioxide (E171) is not safe as a food additive because of potential immunotoxicity, neurotoxicity and genotoxicity (meaning it's toxic to our genes and therefore to the next generation).[28] Titanium is easy to avoid, however, by refusing to buy artificially whitened foods or synthetic skincare products, and by using safe, natural toothpastes like those made by Green People. Read the ingredients list on everything!

There are also toxic metals used, worryingly, in medicine: **Gadolinium (Gd)**, used in cardiac scans, may affect the kidneys in vulnerable patients, **Thallium (Tl)**, radioactive and very toxic, is also used in cardiac scans, as is **Technetium (Tc)**, also radioactive. In my practice I've seen people become very ill after MRI scans involving gadolinium and after coronary artery investigations involving thallium. The physicians involved, however, told the patients that it was pure coincidence.

If you would like more info about toxic metals, it's worth checking out the website of the Health Education and Research Trust, www.hert.org.uk – go to 'Environmental Medicine' and then to 'Toxic metals'. The website is run by the brilliant researcher and lecturer Dr Rachel Nicoll, to whom I am very grateful for pointing me towards some of the relevant research studies on this topic.

As I said in the introduction to this section, pollutants don't really stay in separate compartments like earth (the lithosphere), water (the hydrosphere) and air (the atmosphere). They get everywhere. So, pesticides, synthetic fertilisers and heavy metals are in the water too, and indeed in the air, but in the next chapter we'll be primarily looking at other toxins that end up in the water, either through negligence or, in some cases, by being quite deliberately put there. So, get into your wetsuit, hold your nose and let's dive in.

CHAPTER THREE

WATER

The rivers are our brothers, they quench our thirst ...
and feed our children.

Ted Perry, *Home*

Water is the stuff of life; our bodies are about 70 per cent water. We need it for drinking and cooking and for washing ourselves, our clothes, our dishes and our homes. Unless you live by a high mountain stream or have a well in your back garden, the chances are that your water comes out of a tap. Providing safe, clean drinking water to millions of people is a very complex operation, with plenty of opportunities for things to go wrong.

The water companies see their main task – after maximising shareholder profits – as removing pathogenic bacteria from the water; that's what they understand by 'safe and clean'. And this is certainly necessary. In 1854 there was an outbreak of cholera in the Soho area of London, which caused hundreds of deaths, and only stopped when radical doctor John Snow removed the handle from the Broad Street pump. He rightly suspected that the water from that particular well was contaminated with something that caused cholera, although he didn't know that the 'something' was a bacterium, *Vibrio cholerae*. It had come from sewage, which was in those days dumped freely into the Thames. (Sewage is, scandalously, again being dumped in our rivers in the UK; more on that later in the chapter.) Once the pump handle was removed, so the contaminated water source was out of action, the deaths stopped. Despite this success, his colleagues and everyone else thought John Snow was nuts; that has been the fate of other pioneering doctors too, like Ignaz Semmelweis. He was a brave obstetrician in Austria back in the 1800s, who noticed that mothers were dying in childbirth when they had been examined by doctors with unwashed hands – doctors who had just come from working in the morgue. He noticed also that the mothers treated only by midwives did not die. He instituted the practice of handwashing against enormous, and from our perspective ridiculous, opposition.

Ever since the late 1800s, European and American governments have been looking for ways to make tap water free of dangerous microbes. Their solution was, and still is, to use chlorine, a powerful disinfectant that does kill most microbes. Let's have a look at its pros and cons.

Chlorine

Chlorine is an element of the halogen class (group 7 of the periodic table), the others being fluorine, bromine, iodine and astatine. It is a toxic, yellowy-green gas, very irritating to the eyes, lungs and skin, as many of us know from swimming in the local indoor pool. It does kill a lot of bad bugs. When the UK added chlorine to drinking water supplies in the early 1900s, deaths from typhoid reduced dramatically. (Typhoid, like cholera, is a severe diarrhoeal infection acquired from contaminated water.) So far, so good. But – here come the downsides.

Not all bugs are killed by chlorine. There was a massive outbreak of *cryptosporidium*, another waterborne diarrhoeal disease, in Milwaukee in 1993,[1] in which 400,000 people got infected. Over 4,000 needed hospital admission and more than 50 died. There were similar outbreaks in Nevada, Oregon and Georgia. The water supply in all these locations in the US was and remains chlorinated, but the chlorine failed to kill the bugs and the checks in place in the system failed to detect the water contamination.

Chlorine has another major drawback. It combines with natural molecules already in the water to form what are known as disinfection by-products, DBPs. Examples include the trihalomethanes (THMs) such as chloroform (which was used as an anaesthetic in the nineteenth century, but abandoned because it caused damage to the heart and liver), the halo-acetic acids (HAAs), chlorite, chlorate, bromate and hundreds more.[2] Unfortunately, many of these are carcinogenic.[3] Bladder cancer and colorectal cancers are the most-often mentioned in the studies on this problem. What can be done about this?[4]

Two things. First, there is another, safer way to kill the bugs in the water supply. It involves a combination of physical filtering and, crucially, ultraviolet light. Ultraviolet light kills bad bugs and results in no disinfection by-products whatsoever. This is what they have been doing for some years in the Netherlands[5] – I wonder why we can't do it here? It makes evolutionary sense to use UV light; the sun has been known for millennia to be the best disinfectant there is. The Dutch are not drinking all these carcinogenic by-products that we are subject to in the UK and the US; there is a campaign that needs to be fought here.

Second, on the individual level, we had better filter our own water. Ideally, even in a chlorination system, the water companies would remove the chlorine (and its by-products) after it had done its disinfection job. But they don't, and they're not about to. So, perhaps frustratingly, it's down to us as individuals to install a water filter in our home.

First choice: a whole-house water filter, so we're not only avoiding drinking the chlorine and DBPs, but also not inhaling them or absorbing them through our skin in the bath or shower. This, of course, is the most expensive. Second choice: a plumbed-in but kitchen-only water filter, so we are at least drinking and cooking with safe water. Third, and cheapest, and really the only option for students and other people who are renting: a counter-top jug filter. We shouldn't have to go to such lengths, of course, paying our water bills and then paying again to make it safe, but I believe we need to for our own health – unless we are going to move to the Netherlands. Installing a water filter is a far better option than buying water in plastic bottles, both for the planet and for your health – water in plastic bottles has been found to be full of thousands of particles of toxic microplastics. And it works out no more expensive.

A good water filter will not only remove the chlorine and its carcinogenic disinfection by-products, but it will also remove most of the other nasties from our tap water, the ones we are going to discuss in the rest of this chapter, and it will also remove pesticides, which make their way from the earth into our water systems. Making brand recommendations is a hazardous business (although I did venture to do so on page 275 of *SAITT*) as brands can change, go out of business, get taken over... But as a general rule, the company should have been making water filters for many years, and should be able and willing to explain exactly how their product works and which chemicals it removes. They should be able to answer your questions and provide references. Many people now favour reverse osmosis (RO) filters, but I'm not so sure as, although they remove pretty well everything, that includes the good minerals such as magnesium and calcium, which you would have to replace through supplementation. It is all a bit of a minefield, but one well worth taking time to explore because, along with eating healthy, organic food, this is the most important way to stay well in our crazy times.

Fluoride

Fluoride, like chlorine, is a group 7 element. The 'ide' suffix means it is in the form of a 'halide', the fluorine atom having gained an electron to become an ion, like chloride (harmless and necessary), bromide (toxic) and iodide (essential). Fluoride is added to the drinking water supply in the US and the Republic of Ireland, but not in mainland Europe. In the UK, it has been in the water supply in Birmingham since 1964, and a few other regions have added it more recently, usually after a fight. Other parts of the UK have successfully refused. However, at time of writing, the British government is planning to put fluoride in the water supply of the whole country. In Chile and in Cuba and in several European countries, fluoride was briefly added in the past, but then removed rapidly when the dire effects on human health became apparent. So, what's going on?

First of all, here is the reason we are given for the artificial fluoridation of our water: it's good for children's teeth. Prevents decay, prevents cavities. Sounds good. The American and British Dental Associations both support this view. They cite studies showing that tooth decay has decreased concomitantly with water fluoridation, but those studies usually fail to control for other factors affecting tooth development, such as dental hygiene, diet and socioeconomic status.[6] They also fail to account for the fact that in countries that decided to take the added fluoride out of their water, such as Finland and Cuba, there was no subsequent increase in tooth decay.[7] Most importantly, numerous studies show that rates of dental decay among children have been falling every bit as fast in the countries that don't add fluoride to their water as in the countries that do.[8]

From the 1960s to the 2000s, dental decay has been declining, including in all European countries, where no fluoride is added to the drinking water; you can see this graphically illustrated in Professor Paul Connett's excellent book, *The Case Against Fluoride*, using WHO data plotted by Professor Chris Neurath.[9] Furthermore, it turns out that, whatever fluoride does to our teeth, it does it by surface contact, not by being swallowed.[10] Therefore, even for those who believe (wrongly, in my view) that fluoride strengthens children's teeth, there is no reason at all to put it in our drinking water.

Pioneering dentist Weston A. Price was astonished to discover, on his visits to many different tribal peoples in the 1930s, that everyone was in excellent health and had perfect teeth. Beautifully aligned, uncrowded, gleaming white teeth with no decay. A dentist or orthodontist among such people would have been gloriously unemployed. Of course, the peoples' diet was natural and unprocessed, and their intake of fluoride (and other pollutants) was zero.

Whether swallowed or applied directly, what fluoride does do to the teeth is to cause something called 'dental fluorosis', patchy discoloration and eventually pitting of the dental enamel. This has been known for many decades; back in the early 1930s scientists were finding severe tooth mottling in areas where the water supply was high in fluoride. In the US, this was probably due to aluminium mining contaminating wells in the local area[11] – aluminium and fluoride attract each other. Through the 1940s, scientists were therefore looking for ways to reduce the fluoride levels in drinking water. More recently, in other parts of the world where the water fluoride level is too high (due to naturally occurring geology in parts of China) health organisations are, again, making efforts to reduce the fluoride levels in the drinking water because the high fluoride level is lowering IQ[12] as well as mottling teeth. Yet now, this tooth mottling and pitting, not to mention lowered IQ and other hazards we'll discuss below, seems to have been calmly accepted as the price we pay for the decrease in caries that – allegedly – goes along with it.

Fluoride is not a nutrient; our bodies don't need it. Administering it to the populace is not correcting any deficiency. Tooth decay is not caused by a lack of fluoride, but by excess sugar and by failure of tooth-brushing. But that is too simple for Big Business, who prefer complicated and profitable solutions. (More anon on why adding fluoride to our water is so very profitable, and for whom.) Fluoride in fact functions as an anti-nutrient, in that it pushes iodine out of the body, causing harm to the thyroid gland and other organs. So, let's take a look at the damage fluoride does to our bodies and brains, and then we'll briefly examine the real reasons why this stuff is in our water supplies – or soon will be, if we don't stop it.

Bones

What fluoride does to the teeth, it does to the bones: skeletal fluorosis. It makes bones denser but also more brittle – more liable to fracture. Hip fracture in post-menopausal women is a particular risk and carries a high (30 per cent) mortality, with long-term disability in most of those who do survive the first year. A study in the excellent journal *Environmental Health Perspectives*, which I'm afraid very few GPs ever read, looked at the relationship between hip fracture rate and fluoride levels in women's urine. Measuring fluoride in the urine is important; if you just look at how many parts per million of fluoride are in the drinking water, you don't allow for how much water individual people drink; an athlete, for example, will drink far more than average, as will a diabetic, thus increasing their fluoride intake. (And that's apart from all the fluoride that's in conventional toothpaste, dental floss, dental drops, mouthwash and tea. Safe, fluoride-free versions of toothpaste, floss etc. are discussed in chapter 7.)

The study found that women in the highest third of fluoride consumption had a 59 per cent increased risk of hip fracture.[13] This was despite the fluoride level in their water being below the WHO's maximum limit of 1.5 mg/L (milligrams per litre), a limit that, like so many official 'safety' limits, is set way too high. A similar study, from 2021, found a 50 per cent increase in hip fracture rate among women with the highest fluoride exposure, although, again, the water they were drinking was supposedly within safe limits. As well as increased fracture rate, these women had slightly *increased* bone mineral density (BMD), which is meant to be protective against such fractures, but clearly isn't.[14]

In England, there are 65,000 hip fractures annually. Public Health England (PHE), recently renamed the UK Health Security Agency, did a study about this as well. They found a link between water fluoridation and hip fractures, but then claimed that their own results were 'inconsistent'. Indeed, they were, and we'll see why shortly: serious methodological flaws, leading to an underestimate of the impact of fluoride on hip fracture rate. Professor Chris Neurath, of the American Environmental Health Studies Project and the Fluoride Action Network in the US, and Penelope Sowter in the UK, asked PHE for their raw data to analyse; this is the civilised way to do research scholarship, by sharing data.

But PHE refused to release this information, and even refused to name their report's authors. So instead, Neurath and Sowter used publicly available data on fluoride levels and hip fracture rates in different areas of England, some of which have fluoride added to the water (as of 2023, most still don't). They took into consideration the important confounding variables that PHE had failed to control for (hence their 'inconsistent' results): poverty in the elderly, ethnicity and water hardness. These factors all independently affect hip fracture rate, and so must be controlled for, in order to get a meaningful result. Having accounted for those factors, Neurath and Sowter found that fluoride levels of just 0.7 mg/L in the water were associated with a more than 20 per cent higher rate of hip fractures. And, for the statisticians among you, the findings were highly statistically significant.[15]

Fluoride distorts bone architecture, and fractures are not the only outcome. There is some evidence, hotly contested, that fluoride increases the risk of osteosarcoma, a very serious and often fatal form of primary bone cancer, mostly occurring in young adults. This had been suspected since the 1950s, from both animal and epidemiological studies, but a definite relationship was found in a study by Dr Elise Bassin at Harvard, showing that boys exposed to fluoride at certain key stages of childhood development had a five- to seven-fold increased risk of getting osteosarcoma by the age of twenty.[16] This study was suppressed for years and its findings denied and contradicted by Dr Bassin's own 'research sponsor', in a saga of shocking corruption thoroughly documented by Professor Paul Connett.[17] Dr Bassin concludes her study, as so many academics do, with a call for more research, but somebody has to fund research, and remarkably little has followed on this crucial question.

And now I have to confess to a personal interest in this issue. I lost a very dear friend when we were both twenty-one. She died of osteosarcoma. She grew up in Birmingham and, as I now know, had been drinking fluoridated water from the age of seven. I remember her courage and her suffering, the uselessness of the gruesome treatments she endured and the relentless march of this terrible cancer. I have learnt a lot since, that I wasn't taught in medical school. Perhaps it is because of Nickie that I care so much.

The Brain and Nervous System

In many dozens of studies, fluoride (at the levels added to drinking water) has been shown to be a neurotoxin. These studies include 'meta-analyses' and reviews that look at many other studies combined.[18] Let's start at the very beginning – with the baby in the womb. If there's fluoride in the water, there's fluoride in the pregnant woman and in the amniotic fluid that surrounds the foetus.[19] Babies who are bottle-fed are much more at risk because formula is reconstituted with tap water; all babies have their IQ lowered by fluoride in the water, but the effect is much stronger in bottle-fed babies.[20] In this, as in so much else, breastfeeding is protective.

The higher the prenatal fluoride exposure, the poorer the cognitive outcome; the children have lower scores on tests of mental functioning at any age between four and twelve.[21] Some studies show that the IQ-lowering effect of fluoride intake during pregnancy affects boy babies far more than girls;[22] we don't know why. In Mexico, the fluoride intake is from fluoridated salt, not water, but it does the same damage.[23] Children's brains just do not develop properly if they are exposed to fluoride, whether in the womb or later in childhood.[24] This is not just a loss for those children and their families; it has huge implications for society as a whole. That's a large cohort of tomorrow's adults that contains far fewer gifted people and far more with serious learning disabilities. Sometimes these cognitive deficits due to fluoride exposure are politely called 'developmental delays',[25] but 'delay' implies the children might catch up later. They don't. ADHD (attention deficit hyperactivity disorder) is extremely common among children these days, you may have noticed. It turns out that one of the contributing factors is exposure to fluoride while still in the womb.[26]

The Rest of the Body

Fluoride damages the kidneys[27] and it also affects glands such as the thyroid and pineal. It is associated with underactive thyroid[28] (very common these days and not always diagnosed), particularly in pregnant women. This may well be because, as mentioned above, fluoride is an 'anti-nutrient' that can displace iodine, which is essential for the thyroid gland to make its hormones. Indeed, it has been found that, where there is pre-existing iodine-deficiency, the effects of fluoride on children's intelligence will be even worse.[29] Conversely, fluoride will tend to create iodine deficiency. On the plus side, I have treated fluoride toxicity successfully with iodine, as we'll see in the case history that follows.

The pineal gland, in the brain, has the job of making melatonin, the hormone that helps us go to sleep at night. Its function is interfered with by bright light too late in the evening (as in looking at screens) but also by fluoride, which accumulates in the pineal gland in extraordinary amounts and thereby interferes with production of melatonin.[30] Melatonin is not only required for normal sleep, it also has a role in sexual development and prevents puberty from occurring too early in girls. So, it is possible that, by its action on the pineal gland, fluoride is contributing to the epidemic of premature menarche (periods starting too early) in some countries.[31]

I suspect fluoride damages every other organ in the body too, but if nobody does the research, and independently funded research at that, we won't have definitive evidence. Much of the 'research' purporting to show that fluoride is safe turns out to have been funded by the industries involved in its production, including the aluminium industry.[32] However, from what we know already, the application of the Precautionary Principle would seem to be in order – we need to stop consuming this poison ASAP.

One of the biochemical mechanisms by which fluoride does its damage is by breaking hydrogen bonds. These bonds are essential to the structure of proteins,[33] including enzymes, so, when fluoride is introduced, metabolic pathways are compromised and enzymes don't work. Hydrogen bonds are equally vital for holding the strands of our DNA (chromosomes) together. If the DNA that constitutes our genes gets disrupted, havoc will follow: infertility, birth defects and cancer. That's just basic biology.

Furthermore, the fluoride added to water supplies tends to bring toxic metals along with it: arsenic, aluminium and lead. We've seen in chapter 2 what they can do, even when not combined with fluoride. But remember: a water filter and a good dietary intake of iodine (from fish and/or seaweed) will largely protect you from fluoride. Rory's mum didn't know this; let's see what happened to him.

RORY'S STORY

In my clinic I have seen children (and adults) from all over the UK and Europe, but it took me some years to notice that I was seeing quite a disproportionate number of children with developmental disorders of brain and bone from the West Midlands and Birmingham area and the Republic of Ireland, areas with fluoride added to the water supplies. Rory was one of these; he was nine when his mum brought him to see me from Birmingham, and he had been sent 'round the houses' in search of a diagnosis.

Rory's walk was very strange; I'm not an expert on gait analysis and I couldn't put my finger on it, but let's say his walk was somewhere between a waddle and a stagger. He couldn't run, jump or hop. The paediatric rheumatologist and orthopaedic surgeon whom he'd seen couldn't nail it either. He didn't fit the categories of juvenile arthritis, knock knees, club foot, congenitally dislocated hip or anything else they could name. He didn't have a diagnosis of bowlegs either, although it did look rather like that to me. X-ray results were 'inconclusive', their letters said.

To be on the safe side, I checked his vitamin D level, which hadn't been done in all the rounds of outpatient clinics. His vitamin D result was 25 nmol/L (nanomoles per litre; normal range is 75–200 nmol/L), low enough to have an impact on the immune system and brain function, but not quite low enough to cause rickets, which was an obvious possibility. Of course, I prescribed a vitamin D supplement and maximal sunshine exposure, but I also tested his urine for both fluoride and iodine. Fluoride was sky-high, way over the upper limit that even American labs set, and their levels are set too high because they are used to seeing high levels from people drinking the fluoridated water in the US (an example of confusing what's average or 'normal' with what's healthy). Rory's iodine level, by contrast, was almost zero. This would have impacted on his brain function and on his thyroid function; he was generally sluggish and a bit overweight, both symptoms of low thyroid.

Rory's neurodevelopment was a hard problem. He could read and write – just – but his reading and writing were slow, as was his speech. Arithmetic was very difficult for him too. Rory had a lot of special help at school, but the school's efforts were somewhat hampered by the lack of a clear diagnosis.

It wasn't autism, the paediatric neurologist had said, and it wasn't dyslexia 'as such' (whatever that meant) and it wasn't dyspraxia (although he was very clumsy, and 'dyspraxia' is just a word derived from the Greek for 'clumsy') – there was a long list of things that Rory hadn't got. In the end, they settled for 'global developmental delay'. They never found a name for his weird bone structure and strange walk.

Of course, I improved Rory's diet and I gave him vitamin C for general detox, liquid B vitamins to wake up his brain and zinc plus a little selenium for an immune boost and because the thyroid gland needs them. But the most important intervention was giving him iodine, daily for a few weeks and then twice a week for long-term maintenance. (I cannot discuss the dose I used; you need to work with a practitioner to do this safely. It is possible to overdose with iodine, although it is far commoner to underdose. More info on iodine in *SAITT*.) I re-tested Rory's urine at our third consultation six months later and the iodine level had improved a lot, but not normalised. Why not? Because his mum hadn't put in place the other most important intervention, which was to buy a water filter. Therefore, although his fluoride level had gone down somewhat (thanks to the iodine) it had not gone down into the 'safe' range (though in my view that would be zero), for the same reason.

At this third consultation, finally, Rory's mum agreed to get a plumbed-in water filter. She wanted to help him, of course, but the water filter idea just seemed very alien to her. Indeed it is – we shouldn't need to do it! At our fourth consultation, the penultimate one, nearly a year after the first visit, she had installed a filter, had continued the iodine and other treatments and had noticed a substantial improvement in Rory's cognitive abilities. So had his teachers. He seemed to have 'woken up'. His reading and writing sped up, his speech became far more normal and his arithmetical abilities improved noticeably. His urine iodine was normal, and the fluoride was gone.

I wish I could tell you that his orthopaedic problems resolved as well, but they didn't; whatever had happened to his bones, and possibly to his connective tissue, appeared to be irreversible. I recommended physiotherapy to improve his mobility, and that was all I could do, but I heard from his mother subsequently that his mental functioning continued to improve.

Why Fluoride?

Now to the burning question: if fluoride is so toxic, why is it being added to drinking water? The answer still shocks me, although I have known about it for many years. The form of fluoride that is added, hexafluorosilicic acid (chemical formula H2SiF6, that's 6 atoms of fluoride per molecule), is a waste product of the phosphate fertiliser industry. We learned about synthetic fertilisers in chapter 1, how they damage the soil and weaken the plants, and pollute waterways by causing 'algal bloom'. And we saw in chapter 2 how they are often contaminated with heavy metals. Well, they do more than that.

Back in the 1950s, the fertiliser manufacturers were forbidden to release their toxic waste gases, silicon tetrafluoride (SiF4) and hydrogen fluoride (HF) from factory chimneys, or to release them into rivers or the sea. These gases were known to be dangerous; cattle and crops died downstream from where they were released. So, the industry had a waste disposal problem. They 'solved' it with a technology they call 'wet scrubbers'. These devices capture the toxic gases and mix them with water, resulting in the production of hexafluorosilicic acid, H2SiF6. This process does indeed prevent the gases from being released into the atmosphere. But then what happens? The resultant H2SiF6, still classified at this point as hazardous waste, is packed up into barrels and sold to local authorities to put in their water supply. Then, it is mysteriously reclassified as a 'water treatment' – not as a drug, though, because then it would be legally subject to safety tests. But there are none.

The phosphate fertiliser companies are laughing all the way to the bank. They are not even paying people to take their toxic wastes away; they're being paid for them! I've looked at some of their websites; they've changed the term 'waste product' to 'co-product' – and so, to its shame, has Wikipedia – and they make out that they are manufacturing the fluoride for the purpose of putting it in water to save children's teeth. But they're not; they're just renaming and selling a toxic waste product. This linguistic slippage is positively Orwellian. As Dr William Hirzy of the EPA Union said in his testimony to the US Senate Committee on the Environment and Public Works on 29 June 2000: 'Putting this stuff in the drinking water is in essence just a hazardous waste management tool. It has nothing to do with dental health whatsoever.' In the US alone, he went on, '200,000–500,000 tonnes of scrubber liquor from the phosphate fertiliser industry is now being managed by putting it into your drinking water system'.

But still, why would any local authorities, national governments or water companies want to buy this junk and put it in the water? One can only surmise that, as with governments' cosy relationships with the pesticide (and fertiliser) companies implied in chapter 1, there is collusion. We tend to think of governments (public, elected) and industry (private, unelected) as two completely different sets of organisations, but that view is sadly outdated.[34] We know that private industries lobby governments intensively; lobbying is a polite word for bribing. Essentially: 'We will give your party loads of dosh if you pass the laws we want, and refrain from passing any that might restrict our activities'. There tends to be a 'revolving door' between government regulatory bodies and the industries they are supposed to regulate; often the same people rotate seamlessly between the two roles. They play both poacher and gamekeeper, and each is familiar with the other's rules and tricks. Where there are vast sums of money involved, there is corruption. Much more on how this works in the case of fluoride in the book *The Fluoride Deception* by Chris Bryson,[35] formerly of the BBC.

But the phosphate fertiliser industry, it turns out, is not the only industry involved in this. Apart from the dental industries that sell products like toothpaste, mouthwash, toothpicks and dental floss all contaminated (sorry, 'enhanced') with fluoride, and the professional dental associations that seem to be in industry's pocket (although most of their rank-and-file members are probably innocent true believers), there is another piece of this scandalous puzzle. Who else might have a strong interest in pretending that you could prevent tooth decay just by putting something in the water? Why, the industry that causes tooth decay, of course! The sugar industry – we could call it 'Big Sugar' – is huge and powerful and has always been in the business of propagandising to try to convince us that sugar is harmless (see *SAITT*, page 24). They have spent many decades buying up academics and government officials to promote the line that sugar is good for us and that fluoride is safe and effective.[36] So, we get two poisons for the price of – our health. This is all very profitable. It is forced mass 'medication' (except that fluoride is not a medicine by any definition) without informed consent, in fact without any consent, without even our knowledge. Some would say it's an infringement of our human rights, and against the Nuremberg Code.

Plastics: The Final Straw

Plastics are poisonous. They're poisoning the rivers, the oceans, the air, the earth and us. Plastics are synthetic polymers, long chain molecules that do not biodegrade. Once used, we throw them away – but it turns out that there is no such place as 'away'. In landfill, plastics break down into smaller and smaller bits until we have microplastics, finding their way into the groundwater, then the rivers, then the sea, then the fish, then us. This physical breakdown into microplastics is not the same as biodegrading. In biodegradation, as happens to the cabbage leaf on your compost heap, the thing is turned into something else entirely, by natural processes. Some optimistic scientists are currently bio-engineering bacteria to be able to biodegrade plastics, but I'm not holding my breath; it was high tech that got us into this mess and I doubt that high tech will get us out. What will get us out is more or less ceasing the production of plastics – and that means that we, the public, have to stop buying them, particularly the single-use plastics.

There is some good news now: public awareness of the problem of plastic pollution is growing rapidly. We may well have seen, by the time this book goes to press, the production of the very last plastic straw. May it be followed speedily by the last ever plastic bag – and here again, we have seen great progress in recent years. But before I tell you the story of some successful campaigns against plastic, I need to tell you how there came to be so much of it about, and why it is a problem, for our bodies as well as for the planet as a whole.

I first heard the phrase 'The Tyranny of Convenience' from Nick Barnard of Rude Health, at the Groundswell agricultural conference in June 2021. It's also the title of an article by Professor Tim Wu, from the *New York Times*, 16 Feb 2018. It's relevant here because plastic, invented in 1907 and already being mass produced by the 1940s, is very convenient indeed. We carry water in it, store food in it, keep cleaning chemicals in it, make toothbrush handles out of it, line tins with it, make kiddies' toys with it, stir coffee with it, go fishing with it and wrap just about everything in it. Supermarket foods are packaged in it, vinyl floors and furniture are made of it, 'personal care' products and air 'freshener' sprays are full of it.

However, we can carry water in glass bottles or metal or bamboo containers, store food in ceramic dishes, ditch the cleaning chemicals entirely (how and why are explained in chapter 7), buy toothbrushes with bamboo handles (from companies such as Woo Bamboo), stop eating tinned food (which is rubbish anyway), give our kids toys made from real, natural materials like wood (or let them play with whatever's around, like pots and pans, and create their own games, as they always used to), stir our coffee with real spoons and rediscover the joys of the brown paper bag. Fishing tackle I know nothing about, but I do know that humans have been catching fish for thousands of years, since long before plastic was invented, so it must be perfectly possible to fish without the plastic bits and bobs. This matters quantitatively, as the number of 'recreational anglers' in the UK is in the millions. If they all stopped using plastic tackle, that would be a whole lot less plastic eventually ending up, via landfill, in the sea, where – guess what – it poisons fish.

Returning to our list, floors and furniture can be made of natural materials, alternatives to toxic 'personal care' products and air 'fresheners' are discussed in chapter 7, and I'll return to supermarket packaging later in this section.

I've suggested quite a few changes here – but why should we make them? Why should we go to such lengths to break 'The Tyranny of Convenience'? Because a boycott of plastic products will cut the problem off at source. We can do this, and two wonderful, practical, short, simple and eminently readable books can help us do it: *How to Give Up Plastic* by Will McCallum of Greenpeace[37] and *How to Save the World for Free* by Natalie Fée.[38] Greenpeace are doing great work on this issue. And see also the incredible organisation that Natalie Fée has created, www.citytosea.org.uk.

I remember when you would return a bottle (glass or plastic) to the shop and get 10 pence back. This sort of incentive scheme would be easy to reintroduce, with a more substantial proportion of the price being effectively given as a deposit at purchase and reclaimed when returned. If you are shopping online, the delivery person could take back the plastic bottles and the money be taken off your bill. There is an added urgency for the public and the government to insist that shops and supermarkets do this; plastics are not only toxic in themselves, they are made from fossil fuels, so their manufacture contributes mightily to the release of toxic air pollution and climate chaos as well as choking the oceans with plastic litter. Of course, it's good to reuse or at least recycle, but it's so much better not to make/buy the stuff in the first place. Stuff – we don't need so much STUFF! The sum of human happiness would not, I believe, be diminished one iota if no plastic ducks or plastic flowers or plastic baubles were ever produced again.

And besides, recycling isn't always what it appears to be. As shown in Channel 4's recent Dispatches documentary, *The Dirty Truth about Your Rubbish*, a lot of what we conscientiously put in our recycling bins in Britain is not being recycled at all.[39] Many local councils are so strapped for cash that they chuck half of it into incinerators, so we end up inhaling microplastics and other toxic by-products of the burning. Or they ship it off to poorer countries, paying them to take our crap and spreading the plastic poison – which lasts for centuries – across the planet. Neocolonialism.

The Plastic inside Us

Here's the low-down about what plastic does to our bodies. The 'plasticiser' substances used to make plastic flexible (the word plastic means malleable or flexible) are the lethal and almost unpronounceable phthalates. They interfere with our metabolism and lead to a significant rise in the incidence of diabetes. They are endocrine disruptors, causing substantial weight gain, just like pesticides. Anyone dieting and exercising heroically yet failing to shed their excess fat might want to stop wrapping their food in clingfilm (plastic wrap), stop drinking anything from tins (lined with plastic) or plastic bottles and stop using synthetic moisturiser/make up/ perfume/deodorant, which all contain microplastics (safe alternatives are mentioned in chapter 7), as well as eating organic food and filtering their water to remove the microplastics along with other toxins.

Phthalates leak into food from the plastic packaging around it.[40] High levels of phthalates measured in people's urine have been associated with infertility, endometriosis, delayed puberty (in both sexes) but premature breast development, sperm damage, cancer, thyroid damage and even allergies, asthma, eczema, psoriasis and depression.[41] I can't help thinking of the little boy who was brought to see me, his mum distraught because he was growing breasts. He was eight. His GP had said, extraordinarily, 'Oh don't worry, man boobs are quite common among the youngsters these days.' Indeed, they are, but personally I think that represents potentially serious underlying problems. I tested the little boy and his mum, and their urinary phthalate levels were through the roof. She had been a real plastic junkie from well before he was conceived; plastic water bottles, clingfilm, air freshener sprays, synthetic perfumes, the lot. But so are we all, unless we happen to have learned how dangerous the stuff is. I had to spend a lot of time assuring her that it was not her fault; you cannot act on knowledge you don't have. This mum changed her lifestyle dramatically, and her own health improved, and I did manage to detox the phthalates out of the little boy's system. The boy boobs didn't disappear, but they did stop growing. (This consultation, by the way, was carried out with utmost discretion, the little boy thinking it was a general health check; nothing was said in his presence to make him feel bad about his body.)

Bisphenol A (BPA) is a very common plastic chemical, found in the linings of tins, including tins of baby food, baby's bottle teats, cigarette smoke, till receipts and as a contaminant of packaged, processed food. It is a neurotoxin, implicated in neuroblastoma,[42] a brain cancer that used to be very rare but is getting more common year on year. BPA is also an endocrine disruptor. It's oestrogenic, meaning that it stimulates oestrogen receptors, feminising male mammals and fish, contributing to breast and prostate cancer and to polycystic ovary syndrome (PCOS).

Another endocrine effect of BPA is on the thyroid gland. It interferes with the conversion of one form of thyroid hormone, T4, into the more active version, T3.[43] I have lost count of the number of patients I have seen who have all the features of an underactive thyroid gland – fatigue, constipation, weight gain, dry skin, dry hair, puffiness, sluggish brain and more – who have been told that their thyroid hormone level is normal. But on further enquiry it almost always transpires that only T4 has been measured, not T3. When I test, I find that T4 is not being converted into T3, even in people who are not genetically prone to this problem, and who are not deficient in the nutrients needed for this conversion (selenium and zinc). I can treat this with tiny doses of T3 or, preferably, with natural desiccated thyroid hormone, but why is it happening? In these cases, it seems that BPA from plastic is a likely culprit.

BPA is also strongly implicated in our obesity epidemic. How does BPA contribute to obesity? It's all about hormonal signals, and not just thyroid. Feeling full up after a meal is down to the balance of two hormones in the hypothalamus in the brain. They are called leptin and ghrelin; leptin tells you that you're full and ghrelin tells you that you're still hungry. BPA damages the leptin receptors in the hypothalamus, which messes up this balance; you don't get the leptin message. This leads to people feeling hungry all the time. They have no sense of satiety, even after a good meal. This is so important; I really don't believe that a quarter of our population have suddenly become greedy gluttons. I believe they're being poisoned, not only by sugary drinks, junk food and inactivity but also by plastic toxins like BPA and phthalates.

BPA is also implicated in kidney disease, prenatal exposure to BPA is linked with childhood asthma,[44] and urinary levels of BPA are strongly linked to incidence of heart disease.[45] BPA has also been linked with autoimmunity;[46] autoimmune diseases are becoming more and more common these days and include rheumatoid arthritis, multiple sclerosis, lupus, Crohn's and Hashimoto's. In fact, I can't think of a single body system in which BPA isn't doing serious damage.

Now we know all this, we'll want to avoid BPA and similar chemicals, of course. But we have to be a bit cautious here. The manufacturers, like all profiteers, are quite clever. They know we're getting worried. So, you may now see a product advertised as 'BPA-free!' – but don't get too excited. Usually, they have just replaced bisphenol A with another bisphenol. But I predict, based on experience of how chemical companies behave, that bisphenols B–Z will prove to be similarly toxic. Avoidance of plastic is the safest way.

All these toxins are too much for the poor old liver, doing its best with a demanding detoxification schedule it wasn't evolved to cope with. So, now we have a new disease, 'Non-Alcoholic Fatty Liver Disease', or NAFLD, and specifically 'Toxicant-Associated Fatty Liver Disease', or TAFLD.[47] BPA and the phthalates are bad for our gut microbiome too, but the flip side of that is that taking probiotics (healthy gut bacteria in a capsule or fermented foods like kefir, kimchi and kombucha) can protect you somewhat. Probiotics reduce the absorption of these chemicals, as they do that of heavy metals.[48]

Further good news is that, although BPA is toxic, it is not persistent. It leaves the body within 6–24 hours. So, all we have to do to get rid of it is to stop taking it in. No elaborate detox regimes required; just stop eating/drinking it or slathering ourselves with plastic-infested 'personal care' products. Yet over 90 per cent of Americans have BPA metabolites in their urine[49] (metabolites are the result of the liver's heroic efforts to detox the substance), especially people eating tinned food (tins are lined with BPA-containing plastic).

Taking It Back

Do you remember the amazing shepherdess Rebecca Hosking from chapter 1? She is also a heroic anti-plastics campaigner. She was the lead photographer and co-producer of the 2007 BBC film *Message in the Waves*, which you can still watch on YouTube. What she saw in the remote Pacific Ocean was profoundly shocking. Baby albatrosses, who normally eat squid and other brightly coloured marine creatures, were eating plastic instead. The parent birds were feeding it to them in all innocence; it looked like their usual food. All that coloured plastic in the ocean around Midway, an isolated Pacific Island 1,000 miles west of the main Hawaiian archipelago; the chicks were eating it and dying. The plastic bits we threw away ended up in the stomachs of these beautiful, precious birds. Two years later, in 2009, photographer Chris Jordan documented the identical nightmare scenario. In 2017, Sir David Attenborough made a film showing the same tragedy, as part of the *Blue Planet II* series.

So, Rebecca came back to her home town of Modbury in south Devon, and started the campaign against plastic bags. Modbury was the first town in Europe to go plastic bag-free, and also to stop using plastic cups, plastic cutlery and so on. All the shopkeepers there watched her film and shared Rebecca's grief about the albatrosses, and also the dolphins and seals who were all tangled up in our discarded plastic. They all agreed to change to bags made of corn-starch, paper or cloth. It can be done! Within three or four months, 130 other UK towns had gone plastic bag-free or pledged to do so. Then all thirty-three London boroughs followed. The then-prime minister Gordon Brown was so impressed that he brought in the tax on plastic bags, initially 5p, then 10p, and the next prime minister, David Cameron, implemented it.

This is one example of what can be achieved. Another is the impressive work of ClientEarth, a group of concerned lawyers who challenge governments on the illegal damage they are doing, or allowing to be done, to our planet. They are taking the food company Danone to court over the massive plastic pollution the firm has caused globally; do look up ClientEarth and support them. There is much to be done politically and through the courts, as well as avoiding the use of plastic products in our own lives, as described in the two books mentioned above.

I have a fantasy about supermarket packaging. Yes, really, I do! Imagine the following. You go shopping and you buy fruit and vegetables, cheese, nuts, beans, rice, pasta and loo roll. You get home and notice that it's all wrapped in plastic, the soft plastic that can't be recycled even by a fully functioning local council (if there are any of those left). Normally you would put all that packaging in the bin. But you've seen Rebecca's film, you've read what I've just written or the books by Natalie Fée or Will McCallum – and you've gathered together a group of fifty or so concerned friends and neighbours who all shop at the same supermarket. They're all unwrapping their shopping at home too, but this time they are not binning the wrapping. The next morning, all of you turn up at the supermarket. You have brought all the plastic packaging back – the supermarket chose to use it and now they have to figure out what to do with it because you all dump it on the floor and leave. All fifty of you – and maybe the following week, five hundred of you.

When you return, you give out leaflets about how the supermarket could do things differently. They could adopt the strategy of zero-waste shops: loose loo rolls and rice, beans, nuts, seeds, porridge, fruit and veggies in big containers, and all the customers bring their own small paper bags and large cloth bags to put it in. This is not rocket science, it's just how shopping used to be, and could be again. For customers who have not tuned in yet, and have forgotten to bring bags, they can buy paper or cloth or cornstarch bags there and then. If the supermarket doesn't do what it needs to do, you bring the plastic packaging back again and again, until they get the message and stop using it. It can be done. I'll see you there!

It All Comes Out in the Wash

As an ecological medicine practitioner, my focus has tended to be on nutrition and on how to avoid the toxins that can enter our bodies via our gut from food and drink, and via our lungs from the air. But hang on. The skin is the largest organ of the body! It absorbs toxic chemicals from synthetic perfumes, creams and so on (safe alternatives explained in chapter 7) but also, potentially, from our clothing and our bed linen. Most of the chemicals that contaminate our fabrics are petrochemicals and are lipophilic – fat soluble – so they can penetrate the skin. Then they will head for fatty organs – like the brain. Let's start by looking at the synthetic fabrics that constitute a higher and higher percentage of clothing materials worldwide.

Nylon, polyester, acrylic and so on are not breathable, so can irritate the skin in some people, and manufacturing them (from petroleum) contributes to greenhouse gas emissions. When they're washed, they shed zillions of microfibres. Plastic microfibres. They are a major source of the indestructible microplastics described in the previous section; one third of all the plastic in the ocean is coming from our synthetic clothes![50] These microplastics get eaten by zooplankton and crustaceans, move up the food chain to fish and eventually get eaten by mammals like whales and humans; the plastic pollution that our synthetic clothes are causing comes back to bite us in the form of all the illnesses we've mentioned.

Furthermore, unlike natural fibres, synthetic fabrics are not fire-resistant. So, the manufacturers are required by law to impregnate them with flame retardants like PBBs, polybrominated biphenyls. (Note the word bromine hidden in there. It's a toxic halogen like chlorine and fluoride.) These substances are incredibly nasty, classified by IARC (International Agency for Research on Cancer) as probable human carcinogens. Then there's formaldehyde. Formaldehyde is a dangerous reproductive toxin also classified by IARC as a carcinogen (in a nutshell: anything that damages our DNA will affect both reproduction of people, leading to infertility and birth defects, and reproduction of cells, leading to cancer). What's formaldehyde doing in our clothes? It's making them non-crinkle, non-iron, that's what. All those ultra-convenient non-iron shirts – it's formaldehyde making them that way. Don't buy them. You could choose the less convenient but safer option and iron your clothes; however, if you think life's too short to iron a shirt, you can put your clothes on creased and discover that the creases mostly disappear within a few minutes of wearing.

If the clothes you are about to purchase are conveniently stain-resistant, water-resistant and odour-resistant as well as wrinkle-resistant – stop and take a breath. I'm so sorry to tell you this, but what makes them so is a whole new class of chemicals called PFAs, polyfluoroalkyl substances or perfluoroalkyl substances. Note the 'fluoro' in there; yes, it's fluoride again, lots of it. We'll discuss these 'forever' chemicals briefly in the following section, but for now let's just note that they are carcinogenic and are in about 75 per cent of all waterproof and stain-resistant clothes.[51] You probably won't wear a raincoat directly next to your skin – please don't – but still, when it gets washed and eventually disposed of, those chemicals leach out into the environment and, as we now know, what goes around comes around. And that's without even considering the damage to the health of the people who manufacture, apply and work with these chemicals.

Let's Go Natural

So, let's cheer ourselves up by looking at natural fabrics. Cotton is natural; it's a plant that grows. Yes indeed, and 100 per cent organic cotton is great, and also uses less water to grow than does non-organic cotton. At the moment, only about 5 per cent of the cotton grown globally is organic, although that proportion is rising. Most cotton is still grown using vast amounts of pesticides, herbicides or insecticides. It doesn't have to be: as we saw in chapter 1, Pesticide Action Network (PAN) are supporting some African farmers to grow their cotton organically. The main reason that the good people I spoke to at PAN want us to buy solely organic cotton clothes and bedding is because of the devastating impact of pesticides on the health of cotton workers and their children, and that, of course, is a more than sufficient reason for us to make the change to 100 per cent organic cotton. However, in addition, I am concerned about the invisible, chronic effects of pesticides in non-organic cotton touching our skin for extended periods of time: bedding, nightwear, underwear, tee shirts, jeans and leggings. There isn't any research that I know of specifically on this – who would fund it? – but we saw in chapter 1 what pesticides are doing to us when ingested; there's no reason why these toxic effects wouldn't be happening equally from prolonged skin contact.

You can get 100 per cent organic cotton clothing/bedding if you search. Greenfibres of Totnes do them; so do Frugi (www.welovefrugi.com) of Cornwall, and Fou (www.foufurnishings.com), also of Cornwall. And more and more outlets are appearing; but if you're buying elsewhere, do check that the item is made of 100 per organic cotton, not just 'made with organic cotton', which may be a con. Always look out for the crucial GOTS certification; it stands for Global Organic Textile Standard. Their logo is for clothes and bedding what the Soil Association logo is for food: strict and trustworthy.

It's not just pesticides we need to worry about in our clothes; as the investigative journalist Alden Wicker documents in her recent book, *To Dye For*,[52] many other chemicals are added to conventional clothing in the process of manufacturing. They have effects like those we have encountered already, being implicated in cancer, autoimmune disease and disruption of the reproductive and endocrine (hormone) systems. These chemicals include toxic dyes like the azo dyes. I often used to find azo dyes when I blood tested very sick patients, and usually they seemed to be coming either from bright coloured hair dyes (pink and blue mostly) via the scalp, or from tattoos; I did not realise that they might have been coming from brightly dyed clothing too.

But it is perfectly possible to get clothing coloured only by natural, botanical dyes, often from the same outlets that sell 100 per cent organic cotton products. For example, Mima Natural Colour (www.mimanaturalcolour.com) produce what they call 'slow fashion', natural fabrics hand-dyed with botanical dyes. When the vat of dye is exhausted it can be safely composted because it's only made of plants. And, if you make your own clothes, there are countless books now on how to make your own safe, natural dyes from plants you can grow in the garden. If you dye organic cotton clothes with them, you know that when they finally wear out and have to be disposed of they will safely decompose; they're not going to be adding to the cycle of pollution.

There are other completely natural fabrics besides cotton and, as Amelia Twine, founder of Sustainable Fashion Week, points out, they can be grown in the UK, whereas cotton can't.[53] Linen (flax) and hemp are making a welcome comeback, and you can get clothes, bags and other items made from them. They are durable, safe and sustainable, which is not surprising; we've been wearing them for thousands of years. Amelia says that people are now also making clothes out of stinging nettles – who knew that? – and that the fibre from the nettles is smooth, shiny and comfy, and doesn't sting at all! All these fabrics are harmless to person and planet when they're made, when they're worn, when they're washed and when they're finally worn out.

Wool, of course, is an important natural fabric too, but you want to make sure that the sheep weren't dipped in an OP (organophosphate) insecticide dip. The main reason so many sheep are still dipped, according to regenerative farming expert Russ Carrington, is that 'we have overdeveloped the sheep species away from some of their naturally resilient genetics', making them more vulnerable to fly strike and similar problems. Hot, wet summers and warmer winters as a result of climate change exacerbate this, Russ says, as does the decline in populations of bats and birds who would have eaten up most of the pesky flies.[54]

Rebecca Hosking's sheep are never dipped in insecticide. Her 'forever flock' of multicoloured sheep, traditional breeds that thrived in the UK before the time of the enclosures,[55] produce fine, organic wool that Rosie Anderson, a fellow Devonian, makes into the kind of sheepskin rug that even vegan customers have queued to purchase. Rosie uses felt to make the backing for the rug, not the sheep's own skin; that's why the sheep can live out their full, natural lifespans. And the following year you can get a matching rug from the very same sheep – they each have distinctive colours and patterns. And names. You can lay your baby on one of these rugs secure in the knowledge that the baby won't be absorbing any toxic insecticides through their skin. Rebecca's / Rosie's 'no harm' sheepskins can be found at: www.feltedsheepskins.co.uk.

As awareness about all these problems with fabrics is growing, so is the market for alternatives. Here we enter a bit of a minefield, where it may be hard to tell which brands are genuinely safe and 'green' and which result from a company just jumping on the 'green bandwagon' for commercial reasons. Rayon and bamboo are examples of fabrics that start off natural – made from plant materials – but then are often treated with chemicals in a way that renders them toxic. Tencel is made from eucalyptus; it may be fine, but it may be blended with toxic chemicals – we all have to become researchers to be sure!

The July–September 2022 issue of *Positive News* featured six new materials that are supposed to be safe and sustainable. Allbirds' Tree Flyer trainers are made from SwiftFoam, which is meant to be low carbon and sustainable. Pangaia make clothes out of C-Fiber lyocell, using seaweed and eucalyptus, as well as a material called Kintra, apparently a biodegradable version of polyester. Mylo Unleather from Bolt Threads is made from fungus and used to make vegan 'leather' bags. The company Sympatex are turning plastic bottles into anoraks, and when they're worn out you send them back to be recycled by a company called Worn Again Technologies. Lastly, Vegea are turning the skin, seeds and stems of grapevines into another vegan alternative to leather, called grape leather, which other brands can then use to make shoes and handbags; for example, Lerins make their vegan trainers from it. This all seems to be going in the right direction: watch and see!

Keep It Going

One of the many important things I learnt at Sustainable Fashion Week (SFW) in September 2022 was this: 'Your most sustainable item of clothing is the one that's already in your wardrobe.' Amelia Twine says that there are already enough garments on the planet to clothe the next six generations; that's a scary amount of excess, of waste. In other words, what we need to do with our clothes is to maintain, repair, repurpose, swap, sew, sell and pass them on – anything to minimise the purchase of new clothes. Because every time an item of clothing gets thrown 'away', unless it's made from organic cotton, wool, linen or flax and dyed only with natural, botanic dyes, then it is adding to the planet's – and our own – burden of microplastics and other toxins. There are companies through which you can sell on your old clothes – such as Vinted, Depop, Owni – and companies from which you can hire clothes for a special occasion – such as Loanhood, By Rotation and the Hurr Collective. One company that does all of these things is Wear My Wardrobe Out – www.wearmywardrobeout.com – they rent out preloved party clothes and they will repair, alter or upcycle your old ones.[56]

Another gem I heard at SFW was: 'We want hand-me-down clothes, not hand-me-down toxins.' If we must buy, therefore, let's buy from charity shops. But let's also stop and think twice before taking our own old clothes to the charity shop. Doing this used to give me a warm glow of smug satisfaction – until I learned that most of what we give isn't actually sold here in the UK; it ends up in Africa, undermining the local textile economies, and much of it gets dumped there, adding to the toxic pollution of African countries. Another form of neocolonialism, albeit unintentional. Far better to keep our clothes in circulation as long as possible, by using the options mentioned above. This approach is called, generically, 'Slow Fashion', and it's needed because Fast Fashion is making a major contribution to poisoning the planet, the garment workers and the garment wearers.

There is a really exciting movement taking off, which is all about reconnecting fashion with (regenerative) farming. It's called Fibreshed in the British Isles and Fibershed in the US, where it was founded by Rebecca Burgess, a natural dyer, weaver, activist and educator. The 'shed' bit is 'shed' as in watershed or foodshed: an area of land that defines a natural resource base – where streams converge into rivers, and rivers flow into the sea, or where we grow food to feed a given community. A fibreshed is a 'bioregion' where native fibre plants such as cotton, flax and hemp, dye plants, and fibre animals such as sheep or alpaca, thrive naturally, and where they are farmed in agroecological or regenerative systems as described in chapter 1. Clothing made with a fibreshed approach follows the soil-to-soil model, meaning it can safely be composted to feed the soil at the end of its useful life. There are now regional fibresheds covering the UK and the Republic of Ireland, representing a network of farmers, growers, mills, designers and brands committed to producing regenerative clothing that nourishes the earth while giving people the opportunity to (re)connect with their local landscape and support their local clothing economy through what they wear. And also, of course, the chance to wear clothes that don't damage their health. Find out more from Rebecca Burgess's excellent book, *Fibershed*,[57] and also from www.fibershed.org/affiliate-directory, a map of fibreshed initiatives across the globe.[58]

Tougher Choices?

It is not only clothing that touches our bodies. I was horrified to discover that most menstrual pads and tampons are 90 per cent plastic! Luckily, you can get safe, natural, organic versions made by Natracare, who also do wet wipes that are safe for both you and the planet.

The Women's Environmental Network (WEN) have an excellent section on their website called Environmenstrual (www.wen.org.uk/our-work/environmenstrual). It provides all the information you need to find safe, sustainable products; it even tells you how to make your own reusable pads if you want to. It explains other reusable options too, such as menstrual cups or natural sponges. Conventional tampons are a hazard not only to the health of the woman using them, but also to everyone else, especially if they get flushed down the loo. Natalie Fée says that in the UK 2.5 million tampons, 1.4 million pads and 700,000 panty liners get flushed into our sewers every single day![59] Apparently, in terms of plastic volume, that's like flushing 5.6 million plastic bags down the loo daily. They regularly block the sewers. Binning them is better than flushing, of course, but using the safer alternatives is better still because, even from landfill, these things do find their way into the sea, and from there, as we've seen, the plastic and other chemicals get into the fish and back into us. They also kill birds.

Plastic is not the only toxin found in pads and tampons. In the US, Women's Voices for the Earth (WVE) have done an investigation into what else is in them. Their report is called, cleverly, 'Chem Fatale'. It turns out these products contain endocrine-disrupting fragrances, carcinogenic dioxins and furans, glues of all sorts and more, as well as microplastics – not really what we want to be putting on our most absorptive body surface or inside ourselves. So, it really is worth looking into all the alternatives you can find – on WVE's website if you're in the US (www.womensvoices.org), or on that of WEN in the UK (www.wen.org.uk).

What about babies? Nappies (diapers) are a similar issue, for the baby and the planet. At this point, let's stop and take a breath. Well, I'm certainly stopping and taking a few deep breaths. Because I'm about to tell you, based on info from the wonderful website of WEN, that disposable nappy waste comes to nearly one tonne in weight in each baby's first two and a half years. That's 7 kilogrammes per week. Per baby. Single-use nappies are one of the world's biggest contributors to plastic waste. In the UK, we throw away three billion disposable nappies every year – remember that there is no such place as 'away', though – and they are made of 61 per cent plastic, plus a load of other horrid chemicals.

There's another reason for the deep breath. I mean, this is hard stuff to know, of course, but so is everything else in this book. You are very brave to have read this far – thank you! The other reason is, I'm about to recommend baby-friendly, planet-friendly, reusable, washable nappies, but with a sinking feeling and quite a dose of personal guilt.

I remember the sleepless nights. I remember the exhaustion and the craziness and the impossible multi-tasking of having a new baby. I remember the 'just about coping, just about surviving' feeling of it all. And I confess; I did use disposable nappies. I only knew one family who used reusables – this was a long time ago, and they were ahead of their time – and it was quite beyond me to understand how they managed.[60] How they could even think about the planet at all (we didn't know disposable nappies were bad for the babies too) when they were immersed in the all-consuming, hardest job in the world, taking care of a baby? So, whatever you decide, no guilt, please. You are doing your best. You may be in an impossible situation. What follows is Only If You Can; it's information, not instruction!

There are washable, reusable, safe, non-toxic nappies. WEN's website will tell you about them, and, for those in London, WEN have partnered with Real Nappies for London; you can apply for a voucher worth up to £70 to get you started if money is an issue. BUT. What we really need is a washable nappy collection service, a council-funded (or, more realistically these days, charity-funded) laundry service that picks up your bucket of dirty nappies, takes them away to wash and leaves you a supply of clean ones, once or twice a week. New project, anyone? Because parenthood is tough. And yes, I know our great-grandparents did it (well, let's be honest, our great-grandmothers did it) – but they didn't have a ton of emails to answer and probably weren't juggling job with childcare, and anyway they simply didn't have the tempting, ultra-convenient option of disposables. All any of us can do, in any era, is to do our best.

But if you are washing nappies – or sheets, or clothes or anything else – what are you washing them in? Yes, you guessed it, conventional laundry powders are full of toxic chemicals, bad for your skin and for the planet. Ecover is a reasonable alternative, Suma is better, and I believe I've found the purest one available in the UK; it's called Allavare (www.allavare.co.uk). It's run by a sweet young lad called Ed who says he's 'Taking on Big Laundry'. I wish him luck. I'm using his products myself and am very happy with them. (I should just say, for the record, I have absolutely no financial or other connection with any of the shops or companies mentioned in this book. I am impartial. Any company I mention, I've checked them out at time of writing and think they're sound. But things change and small ethical companies do sometimes get taken over by the Big Bad Guys, so please do your own research to keep up to date! Thank you.)

PFAs: The 'Forever Chemicals' Darkening Our Waters

PFAs stands for per- or polyfluoroalkyl substances. I've taken the title of this section from the 2019 film, *Dark Waters*. A picture is worth a thousand words, and a moving picture is worth ten thousand. It's billed as a 'legal thriller', and it documents real events at the town of Parkersburg in West Virginia, USA. In short, the chemical company DuPont were making a particular type of PFAs (there are thousands of types) known as perfluorooctanoic acid (PFOA). They were dumping the resultant effluent at their chemical plant at Parkersburg, where it contaminated the water, leading to cancer, birth defects, other illnesses and many deaths, among people, pets and farm animals.

These chemicals have been manufactured since the late 1940s and their toxic effects have been known secretly to the manufacturers since the 1960s,[61] but were first publicly documented in Callie Lyons' 2007 book whose title says it all: *Stain-Resistant, Nonstick, Waterproof and Lethal: The Hidden Dangers of C8*. The chemical PFOA is also known as C8 because it has a chain of eight carbon atoms, although so do many harmless substances. What makes it lethal is the fluorine atoms (yes, it's fluoride again) attached to the carbon atoms. The chemical bond between carbon and fluorine is so strong, it's effectively unbreakable; that's why these substances last forever, and why the damage will persist for generations in Parkersburg and other affected places, wherever factories making this sort of chemical have been located.

But the risk is to all of us, not just those exposed by occupation or by living somewhere like Parkersburg. PFAs are in Teflon and similar coatings that make pans non-stick, they are in stain-resistant carpets and waterproof clothing. They are in some food packaging, especially takeaway tubs from fast-food outlets and microwaveable popcorn bags, some paints, cosmetics, shampoos, bike lubricant oils and shoes.[62]

PFAs don't have to be mentioned on the label, though. They've been found by chemical analysis to be in many school uniforms,[63] even when the uniforms are labelled '100% cotton' or indeed as 'green'.[64] They're in firefighting foam and in firefighters' uniforms – firefighters have five times the heart attack rate and three times the cancer rate of the general population.[65] Some of that is bound to be due to inhalation of burning plastics, but much of it may also be due to skin contact with PFAs, and indeed from ingesting PFAs if they eat their lunch while still wearing their 'protective' gear.

PFAs damage the thyroid gland[66] and the baby in the womb.[67] They are linked to earlier menopause,[68] which matters because it increases the risk of osteoporosis and other problems for women later in life. They are also implicated as causes of obesity, neurodevelopmental and behaviour problems, raised cholesterol, lowered immunity, asthma and kidney disease.[69] Children are most at risk because of their relatively small mass and high surface-area-to-volume ratio, and because when they're very little they tend to be crawling on the floor, absorbing PFAs from the stain-resistant carpet into their skin – and putting their hands in their mouths.

Diabetes is a major epidemic now, affecting younger and younger people, and a recent study found that, among women in midlife, the concentration of PFAs in their bodies was directly related to their chance of getting diabetes.[70] PFAs also increase the risk of liver cancer,[71] those people with the highest levels in their bodies being 4.5 times more likely to develop liver cancer than those with the lowest levels. (The substance in this study was PFOS, perfluorooctane sulfonate, another type of PFAs; it's all essentially the same stuff). Other studies have connected the PFAs with testicular cancer, kidney cancer, infertility, endometriosis, childhood obesity and more.[72]

They're in the water.[73] In February 2022, residents of the Cambridgeshire villages of Stapleford and Great Shelford in the UK were informed by Cambridge Water that back in June 2021 they'd had to remove a water supply that contained four times the upper limit of PFAs. Probably the PFAs contamination had come from the nearby Duxford airfield, where PFAs might have been used in firefighting foam. Having finally informed the residents, Cambridge Water refused to tell them for how long they had been drinking the contaminated water; they'll probably never know. The upper limit is set by the Drinking Water Inspectorate (DWI). It's way too high, at 100 nanograms per litre, but even that isn't properly enforced. It's not even legally enforceable, says Professor Crispin Halsall of the University of Lancaster.[74] Professor Andreas Kortenkamp, director of the Centre for Pollution Research and Policy at Brunel University, agrees. He says: 'The DWI's current safety limits are far too high. Authorities are failing the UK by not putting pressure on water companies to reduce PFAs levels significantly'.[75]

I would add that when water companies are privatised, as is the case now in the UK, such abuses are virtually inevitable, as we'll see in relation to sewage in the next section. The profit motive trumps everything, and the legal as well as psychological reality is that the companies' top priority is to deliver profits to their shareholders, not safe water to the public.[76]

What Can We Do?

Apart from getting a water filter ASAP, and campaigning for the water supply to be re-nationalised and decontaminated, here are some tips to avoid PFAs:

Cookware: there are plenty of PFAs-free alternatives, and some of them are actually non-stick too; they're detailed in chapter 7.

Waterproof clothing: according to *Which?* magazine, 92 per cent of Patagonia's outdoor gear is totally PFAs-free, and that figure should be 100 per cent by 2025. Paramo and Seasalt are also PFAs-free, and all three brands use organic cotton too. Polartec announced in 2021 that it will eliminate all PFAs from its clothing range. I do hope that's true, but I find it hard to be certain; Polartec are owned by Milliken, who have an appalling record on PFAs pollution.[77] Until the law compels companies to reveal their full 'ingredients list', they can shelter behind 'commercial confidentiality' and we can never 100 per cent know what's gone into their products.

You can buy safe, natural brands of shampoo, cosmetics and so on (more details in chapter 7) and you can avoid plastic packaging and takeaway containers. Avoiding plastic will largely enable you to avoid PFAs.

With regard to wrapping, paper bags from If You Care are a good option. For safe greaseproof paper for baking, the Scottish environmental group Fidra (www.fidra.org.uk) found that greaseproof paper sold by the supermarket Waitrose was free of PFAs, and you can also get safe greaseproof paper from Nordic Paper.

For camping gear and outdoor gear generally, Fidra recommend Jack Wolfskin, Endura and Polartec. They also say 'don't lay artificial turf in your garden' – apparently artificial grass contains PFAs. Real grass is of course far better – so long as you don't spray it with herbicides! Much more info on the latest campaigns and how to stay uncontaminated from www.pfasfree.org.uk.

Chemical companies (including drug companies) do periodically admit, usually after prolonged court battles and fines that seem massive to us but are petty cash to them: 'Oh, sorry, that was toxic. OK, we'll replace it with something else.' Then the 'something else' turns out to be a very similar molecule, with the same damaging effects on people and planet. And it all takes years. But here's an example of a case where campaigning groups refused to let them get away with it. The NGO ClientEarth combined forces with the charity Chem Trust (www.chemtrust.org) to challenge Chemours, a company that is a spin-off from DuPont (of *Dark Waters* infamy). Chemours make 'Gen X' chemicals. These were touted by the company as a safe replacement for PFOA, but they too turn out to damage liver, kidneys, blood and immune system, to cross the placenta (reducing foetal weight) and to be probably carcinogenic. And, like PFOA, they last forever.

So, the EU's chemicals agency, ECHA, placed these toxic 'Gen X' substances in the category of 'Substances of Very High Concern' (SVHC). Chemours didn't like this, so they took the ECHA to court but, with support from ClientEarth and Chem Trust, the court rightly upheld the ECHA's decision to label poison as poison. Ideally, of course, the EU would have outright banned it. But every little helps, and here at least, for a moment, sanity and justice prevailed against the profit-hungry poison-mongers.

Sewage in the Sea

Britain has many thousands of miles of beautiful coastline and some wonderful rivers. Let's take a brief deep dive now – or maybe not. Perhaps you love to go swimming and don't mind cold water – but you might not fancy bumping up against a turd or a used tampon. In 2023, the water companies of England discharged raw sewage into our rivers and seas, on average, 1,271 times a day.[78] That's more than 460,000 discharges per year. The regulators, Ofwat, seem to be asleep at their post. Since the water companies were privatised, in 1989, they 'have paid out a total of £78bn in dividends'[79] and 'not built a single reservoir'.[80] They have also not fixed the leaks in the pipes that allow three billion litres of water to be lost every day. And our water bills keep rising. In June 2023 the government did fleetingly consider re-nationalising the water companies, but quickly backed off, a spokesman saying, in the case of one particular scandal relating to Thames Water, 'This is a matter for the company and its shareholders.'

No, this is a matter for all of us. There are some wonderful campaigning groups kicking up a stink, if you'll pardon the pun, about this issue: check out Surfers Against Sewage (www.sas.org.uk) and River Action (www.riveractionuk.com) and join them if this is the thing that gets you most fired up. Not only are sewage discharges unpleasant and hazardous for human health, they also damage the fish and other aquatic creatures, and cause overgrowth of toxic algae further downstream on the shore, exactly as synthetic fertilisers do, as described in chapter 1. Water is a public good and a public right; it should never have been privatised. This is all about greed. Honestly, I think they would privatise the air if they could.

Drugs on Tap!

We humans swallow prescribed medications, over-the-counter medicines and both legal and illegal addictive drugs. When we pee, these end up in the water supply – so everybody else is taking them too.[81] In really tiny doses, but every day. The fish are taking them too and it is doing them no good.[82] Similarly, when animals on (non-organic) farms are given routine antibiotics, these get peed out onto the ground and flow into the water table and eventually into the reservoirs. Antibiotics are a particular worry because of the potential for resistance, as explained in chapter 1. Even our cats and dogs are often on medications nowadays, with similar effects on the environment and other living beings.

In my view, drugs have to be included among the 100,000+ chemicals that are contaminating our environment, and they are about the only ones that have ever been tested for safety. But crucially, the testing protocols assume temporary treatment, not continuous daily dosing. Among the drugs most commonly found in the world's rivers are carbamazepine (for epilepsy), metformin (for diabetes), paracetamol, nicotine and caffeine.[83] There are anti-inflammatories and analgesics (pain killers) too.[84] These drugs are also in the sewage and, as we have seen, the sewage is being repeatedly spilled into the rivers. I am particularly concerned about the amount of oestrogen being peed out into our water supplies by the huge numbers of women taking the oral contraceptive pill or hormone replacement therapy. Of course, I'm concerned about the effects on these women themselves, too, but that's another story.

Next time you get a medicine from the chemist, look carefully at the name of the drug. An astonishing number of medicine names these days begin with 'flu' – yes, it means there is fluoride in it. We have **flu**oxetine for depression, **flu**conazole for fungal infections, **flu**drocortisone (a steroid with a fluorine atom added), **flu**cloxacillin (an antibiotic with fluoride added),

fluoro-uracil (used to treat skin cancers and other cancers), **flu**phenazine (an anti-psychotic, used for schizophrenia), **flu**ticasone for asthma and grillions more. 'Slow Release' medicines are particularly likely to contain fluoride because, as we've seen, it makes the molecule harder to break down, so it will last longer in the system. One might almost begin to suspect, with so much fluoride swimming around in our medicines (as well as in our water, toothpaste, mouth rinse, dental floss and so on) that somebody somewhere had spare supplies of fluoride they wanted to get rid of.

There are only two solutions I can see to the problem of drugs in our tap water. One, sorry you've heard this before, is please do get a water filter, the best one you can possibly afford. The other, longer-term, solution, is that we need to take – and prescribe – far fewer drugs. For ourselves, for our pets and for farm animals. That means a rather different approach to the practice of medicine (both human and veterinary) and is a topic for another day. Meanwhile, take a deep breath and hold it; we're about to explore the pollution of our (not yet privatised) air.

CHAPTER FOUR
AIR

All things share the same breath – the beast, the tree, the person.
The air shares its spirit with all the life that it supports.

Ted Perry, *Home*

I am seven years old, dancing enthusiastically in a circle of children on the grass. Then I start to wheeze. I run out of breath. I feel as if I'm suffocating. I try to keep dancing, but I can't move. I can't even speak.

I've had asthma attacks before, many of them, but not like this. My dad picks me up and takes me to the GP, who knows us well. He gives me an injection of adrenaline. It is nothing short of a miracle. Suddenly I can breathe. I can speak again and even dance; I do a little jig right there in the surgery. I gaze up in wonder at the GP and make a resolution: I want to do what he just did. I want to work such miracles. I shall be a doctor when I grow up.

I had asthma from age three to age twelve; it vanished soon after we moved from a busy main road to a quieter small one. The episode described above occurred in 1964 and was the worst attack I ever had; I was never hospitalised.

Fast forward forty years. Ella Kissi-Debrah was not so lucky. Born in 2004, she was a healthy, happy child; bright, musical, sporty, good at drama, good at everything, and in love with life. Just before she turned seven and living on the terribly polluted South Circular Road, part of the A406 in London, she developed severe asthma. Three weeks after her ninth birthday, in 2013, this beautiful, innocent little girl was dead, her family heartbroken, while the cars and lorries continued in their endless poisonous trundle round the A406. In Ella's last two years she was hospitalised around thirty times. Her initial death certificate said 'acute respiratory failure' – but not what had caused it.

Ella's mother, Rosamund Adoo-Kissi-Debrah, is a secondary school teacher and a brave, intrepid person who has become a heroic campaigner. With help from Professor Stephen Holgate, an eminent respiratory physician and expert in asthma, she realised that the levels of toxic nitrogen dioxide on the South Circular Road were way above both UK and EU 'safe' limits, and the levels of PM (particulate matter) way above the WHO's guidelines. Long story short, at a second inquest in December 2020 the coroner, Philip Barlow, concluded that air pollution was the cause of Ella's death – and indeed of her asthma – and 'air pollution' replaced 'acute respiratory failure' on the new death certificate.

Ella wasn't run over, but traffic killed her.

Take a breath and dry your tears. I certainly cried while writing this short summary of Ella's story for you. But take heart too. Rosamund and many others have never stopped campaigning in honour of Ella's memory and for the sake of all the other people who have died/lost loved ones/will die/lose loved ones because of traffic fumes. Find out more at www.ellaroberta.org. The current mayor of London, Sadiq Khan, who developed adult asthma while training for the marathon, has met with Rosamund, and Ella's story as well as his own experience informed his decision to try to reduce the poisonous fumes that plague the capital's air; more on that later.

I was the only child in my whole primary school to have asthma. Today, every primary school classroom has a shelf devoted to children's inhalers. In 1964, when I had my dramatic trip to the GP (GPs did medicine then; I didn't need to go to hospital), asthma was uncommon and it was never fatal. In fact, I knew that, even at seven; my parents were able to truthfully reassure me, during an attack, that, although I felt I couldn't get enough air, I actually could, and I'd be ok; I wouldn't die. But today, children do die of asthma. Ella is not the only one. So, what's going on? Air pollution is not new, but it's invisible now, often unsmellable; different from the smogs of the mid-twentieth century. It's even more lethal.

This chapter is about outdoor air pollution. (Indoor air pollution is also a problem, but a rather easier one to solve, and is dealt with in chapter 7). In this chapter we'll discuss which toxic substances are in our outdoor air, where they come from, what they do to us (it's not just asthma by any means) and what the solutions are. But first, I need to give you some numbers. Every year, outdoor air pollution causes at least 40,000 excess deaths in the UK and kills about 7 million people globally.[1] In the EU, air pollution is responsible for 300,000 excess deaths a year.[2] And these numbers, which I suspect are underestimates, tell us about the mortality, but they don't tell us about the morbidity, the miserable burden of ill-health; millions of people living with and suffering from the chronic diseases caused by airborne pollution.

Which Toxic Chemicals Are in Our Outdoor Air?

- Oxides of nitrogen, particularly nitrogen dioxide (NO_2)
- Carbon monoxide (CO)
- Ozone (O_3) produced by the action of sunlight on the other pollutants
- Sulphur dioxide
- Particulate matter (PM) – from brakes and tyres as well as engines
- Polyaromatic hydrocarbons (PAHs)
- Benzene (used as an anti-knock agent in petrol)
- Toluene
- Nitrosamines
- Pentanes
- Hexanes
- Dioxins
- Heavy metals (because fossil fuels are contaminated with them)

Where Do They Come From?

All of these toxic substances result from the burning of fossil fuels, which are:

- Coal
- Petrol and diesel made from crude oil
- 'Natural' gas

The airborne toxins in the list above are produced by all internal combustion engines, including those of ships and aeroplanes. Trains running on diesel, of course, produce pollution too, but they can carry so many people that the amount of pollution generated per person travelling is minuscule compared to the impact if all those people go by car. And as for flying – aircraft fuel, a major source of toxicity, is actually subsidised by the UK government to the tune of £7 billion annually. The UK has not only exempted jet fuel from tax, it also puts no VAT on tickets for domestic flights. Our government is effectively paying the polluter rather than making the polluter pay!

People, therefore, will of course choose to fly from Newcastle to Bristol or from London to Edinburgh because it's so much cheaper than getting the train. Government action could turn this around by making trains (and buses) cheap, green, clean, pleasant, efficient and reliable, so we'd choose the train, fly less and drive less. They could fund this by taxing the airlines properly. Some European countries have already banned domestic flights for journeys that could be done by train in two or three hours, and others are actively considering it.[3] And some companies give their employees extra annual leave if they choose to travel abroad for holidays by train rather than plane.[4] This is an excellent trend; air travel is toxic, as evidenced by the increased level of serious illness among those working at – or living near – airports.[5]

The toxins that I listed come mostly from vehicle exhaust, but also from oil refineries, power-generating facilities, factories, industrial processing plants and municipal incinerators. The list of chemicals is not, if you'll pardon the hideous pun, exhaustive. But it contains the main culprits. You'll notice that carbon dioxide is not on the list; it does indeed come out of vehicle exhaust pipes and from all other forms of fossil fuel combustion, but it's not toxic. Whatever else it's doing, CO_2 is not poisoning us, and the other substances listed here certainly are. All of them.

In addition, pesticides also get into our air, particularly in the countryside, when they are sprayed onto fruit trees or ground crops (see chapter 1), and some of the toxic oxides of nitrogen in our air result from the use of synthetic nitrate fertilisers on farms (see chapter 1, again). Both pesticides and synthetic fertilisers are made from fossil fuels too. Plastics, also made from fossil fuels, often get burnt in giant incinerators when we throw them 'away', releasing the highly dangerous, carcinogenic chemicals called dioxins. The rates of childhood cancer, adult cancer and birth defects among people living near such incinerators are significantly higher than the population average.[6] So, plastics, doing damage when manufactured, are doing even more damage when destroyed. And the microplastics from washing and throwing away synthetic clothing that we met in chapter 3 are, it turns out, in the air too, contributing to lung cancer for sure and quite likely to many other diseases.[7] As Dr Stephanie Wright of King's College London says about this, and it applies to almost all forms of pollution: 'You can't clean it up, so it is about stopping it at source'.[8]

What Do These Toxins Do to Us?

In short, they do everything that smoking does. But we don't give cigarettes to toddlers. Car exhaust pipes, however, are just at the height of a toddler's nose.

As with all environmental pollutants, what airborne toxins do to us is mediated via the 'cocktail effect': we are rarely subjected to just one or two of them, but to dozens at a time. This makes it hard to tease out individual effects, to say that chemical X causes disease Y. There are some instances of this, however. Benzene (in petrol exhaust) is linked specifically to acute childhood leukaemia[9] and classified by IARC[10] as a group 1 carcinogen. Whenever I walk along the street and see a kind, concerned person collecting money for a children's cancer charity and simultaneously see children walking or being pushed in buggies through the fume-laden air, I really wonder what we think we're doing. With the best will in the world, the money we give is only furthering the drug companies' futile but profitable search for another initially-heralded but bound-to-fail magic bullet, while the causes of the disease (which has become massively more frequent in recent years[11]) are right there on the street, being inhaled by the kids, by the mothers, by pregnant women, by the kind charity workers, by all of us. (A painful irony here is that benzene replaced lead as an anti-knock agent in petrol; lead was taken out because it was known to be damaging children's brains.[12])

Most studies on the effects of air pollution on health can't single out one pollutant but describe the effects of the whole toxic cocktail. Nitrogen dioxide and particulate matter (PM), however, feature most prominently. For example, nitrogen dioxide has been shown to cause chronic obstructive pulmonary disease (COPD)[13], which disables hundreds of millions of people worldwide and appears to be rising faster than stroke and heart disease.[14] It is commonest among smokers, but plenty of people who don't smoke get it from air pollution, especially in big cities in parts of the world with no regulation at all. You just might remember an episode in March 2014 when lots of people were wheezing, and cars and pavements in London were coated with a reddish orange dust. We were told it was dust from the Sahara. Apparently, however, only 20 per cent of it was that. The rest was nitrogen dioxide mixed with other pollutants from London traffic fumes.[15]

Particulate matter (PM) needs a bit of explaining. It means tiny particles of, basically, soot, but they can be composed of, and coated with, any number of other toxic chemicals, including all those listed above. Their size is measured in microns. A micron is a micrometre, or one millionth of a metre. A human hair is 100 microns wide; PM 10 is 10 microns or less in diameter, and PM 2.5 is 2.5 microns or less in diameter. Modern fossil-fuel-burning cars emit a higher and higher proportion of these very tiny ones, PM 2.5, and some even smaller ones, nanoparticles – a nanometre is a billionth of a metre. Size matters – at the other end of the size spectrum, the bigger the car, the worse the emissions. And, says transport expert Dr David Janner-Klausner, cars are getting bigger by half a centimetre per year, in Europe.

This progressive decrease in size of the PM is due to catalytic converters; regulators forced the automobile industry to fit these, after a prolonged battle some decades ago, to reduce the emissions of toxic carbon monoxide. But, as with so many well-meaning 'tech fixes', there turned out to be a downside: catalytic converters create more and tinier particles of toxic soot. Another painful irony. And a filter fitted to the engine to trap these particles wouldn't help, because most of them are not actually emitted as particles, but as gases that then, once out in the air, condense to form tiny, solid particles.[16] It is these ultrafine particles that are clogging our arteries and increasing the prevalence and severity of asthma and other even more serious lung diseases.[17]

This is because the smaller the particles are, the deeper they can penetrate into our bodies. They get into the lungs and from there into the bloodstream and thus to every cell and organ of the body. We know that PM pollution is causatively linked to lung cancer and to deaths from both heart and lung disease.[18] It is increasing the death rate from strokes as well as heart attacks[19] and, shockingly, is leading to Alzheimer's disease in children and young adults in our most polluted cities. The authors of one study on this, published in the *Journal of Alzheimer's Disease*, surveyed young people in Paris, Mexico City and Santiago, Chilé. They describe the pathology (caused by particulate matter plus ozone) as 'starting in the brainstem and ... relentlessly progressing in the first two decades of life.' They also describe this pollution causing a 'higher suicide risk in youth'.[20] (I'll discuss the role of pollution in mental illness in Appendix I.) Perhaps most disturbing of all is the finding that when pregnant women inhale traffic fumes, the toxic nanoparticles coated with numerous heavy metals are found in their placentas.[21] These toxins are causing low birth weight, prematurity, miscarriages and stillbirths.[22]

Air pollution stops children's lungs from developing and functioning properly. It also makes them more vulnerable to respiratory infections, and Professor Jonathan Grigg has studied the mechanisms by which this occurs.[23] He is Professor of Paediatric Respiratory and Environmental Medicine at Queen Mary University of London, and gave expert testimony at the inquest into Ella Kissi-Debrah's death. He is also a founder, along with Professor Chris Griffiths, of Doctors Against Diesel (www.doctorsagainstdiesel.uk), a partnership with Greenpeace. Professors Grigg and Griffiths were on the working group that produced an important report in 2016, 'A Breath of Fresh Air',[24] from Queen Mary University London, which recommends phasing out coal, expanding clean air zones, better monitoring of air around schools, hospitals and clinics and retaining the EU's regulations.

Schools are an important part of the air pollution equation. As Sadiq Khan shows in his book, *Breathe*,[25] many of the capital's primary schools are in areas where pollution levels are extremely high; deprived children, whose parents probably don't own a car, are breathing the worst air. Equally, parents who drive their kids to school are contributing massively to the pollution inhaled both by their own kids and the kids who are walking to school.[26] 'Walking Buses', where children walk to school in a supervised group, are a great idea, but it would be even better if they weren't walking alongside polluting cars. The fact is, apart from special educational and religious needs, most people would choose their nearest school – in walking distance – if it were a good or outstanding school. This is where education policy, transport policy and health policy need to be joined up (everything is connected); if every school is a good school, nobody needs to drive to get to a school far away from home.

Another expert, Professor Alastair Lewis of the University of York, has shown, perhaps unsurprisingly, that air pollution is far worse in deprived areas.[27] It is exacerbating health inequalities.[28] Dr Ian Mudway of Imperial College has shown, among much other valuable work, that teenagers from ethnic minorities live in more polluted areas than their white counterparts, and that blood pressure in all teenagers is affected by traffic pollution.[29] Furthermore, it turns out that the 'safe limits' for pollution levels, set by governments, are not safe at all; damage from particulate matter and nitrogen dioxide and other air pollutants has been found even at supposedly low levels of exposure.[30]

The burning of fossil fuels has been poisoning adults and children since Charles Dickens' time, although its nature has changed somewhat. Evidence of the damage done has been presented to the powers-that-be on numerous occasions. In the 1990s, the late Dr Dick van Steenis, then a GP in South Wales, noted that children living near oil refineries and oil-burning power stations suffered vastly more from asthma than did their counterparts in other areas; it was due to the same ultra-fine toxic particles that petrol and diesel traffic creates.[31] His study showed that there was also a greatly increased incidence of cancer, heart attacks, diabetes, severe depression and suicide in the high-asthma zone. On a similar theme, and quoting Dr Steenis's work, Michael Ryan gave a statement to Parliament for a public enquiry in 2006, using data from the ONS (Office for National Statistics), showing a significant excess of congenital malformations and premature deaths in areas downwind of the Ironbridge power station in Shropshire, and in areas of Greater London near waste-burning incinerators.[32] His testimony also showed that local officials had obstructed him at every turn in his efforts to bring these facts to light, and that the Environment Agency had failed shamefully in its duty to regulate harmful emissions of PM 2.5.

In Thailand, in the year 2023 alone, ten million people needed medical treatment for air pollution-related illnesses.[33] It simply couldn't be clearer. Air pollution from burning fossil fuels is causing chronic illness and shortening lives. It is contributing massively to neurodegenerative disease in adults (dementia) and neurodevelopmental disorders in children (cognitive deficits, autism, ADHD). It is leading to cancer, heart disease, strokes and mental illness, and damaging everything from sperm to brain to bladder (it's implicated in bladder cancer) to bone (it's implicated in osteoporosis) to skin (it's implicated in acne).[34] And it's massively increasing the burden on the NHS.[35]

The evidence is overwhelming – in two senses. It's overwhelming in sheer volume: 60,000 studies, of which over half have been published in the last ten years.[36] And, of course, it's overwhelming emotionally; as with most of the information in this book, it would, on one level, be far easier not to know it. However, if we don't know, we can't change it. If we do, we can. So: let's talk about solutions.

What Is to Be Done?

I'll give a short answer and a longer answer.

The Short Answer

Fossil fuels, the hydrocarbon remains of plants and animals that died hundreds of millions of years ago, need to be left where they belong, in the lithosphere: the rocky crust of the earth, or deep under the ocean bed. Instead of digging them up and sending them up in smoke, we – humanity – need to learn to manage with safe, non-polluting, renewable alternatives such as solar, wind, wave and tidal power. But how? Partly by stopping all unnecessary uses of energy. To give three examples at random:

1. Leaf blowers on our streets are using up fossil fuels, making a lot of noise and smelly pollution, when a simple, old-fashioned broom would do the job rather better.
2. Large shops have their lights on all night – why? That's using a lot of electricity needlessly.
3. At home; we expect to dress as if we're on the beach. If we put on a jumper, we could turn the heating down a notch or two.

It won't be easy, though, which is why it needs a longer discussion. It may be a case of lifestyle versus life itself.

The Longer Answer

I'll describe an ideal scenario, then the obstacles to that. I'll then briefly survey some recent practical attempts to clean up our air, what the objections to them have been and how they might be resolved. And lastly, I'll list for you (in the Resources section at the end of the book) the numerous amazing organisations that are working to combat air pollution and save our health, so you can see if one of them tugs at your heart strings – or lung strings.

Here's a vision for, let's say, 2040. Children are playing outside, in a city. Most areas are pedestrianised and full of grass and trees, bushes and benches, swings and slides. In those areas that are not, the vehicles are primarily bicycles, in their own lane, and in another lane are a few electric vehicles for the emergency services, disabled drivers, garbage lorries and people like plumbers and electricians who need a van for their work. There are some emergency taxis too, also electric, for anyone who needs to get to a sick relative at short notice. It is pleasant to walk along these city streets because there are no traffic fumes and there's very little noise – electric vehicles are quiet. The pavements (sidewalks) are wide and smooth and well-maintained so that pushchairs (buggies) and wheelchairs can navigate them seamlessly. There are electric buses too. They are mostly 'hail and ride', so you don't need to get to a bus stop. There are delivery lorries too, but only a few and they don't have to go far, because we have become locavores (see chapter 1) – most of what we eat and wear has been grown or raised within a few miles of where we live. The majority of freight is now taken by train, and the trains are electric, not diesel.

The buses are frequent, reliable, cheap and clean, and the driver is not on his/her own; each bus has a conductor too, because nobody should have to work on their own all day long, and the passengers feel (and are) more secure with two staff on board. The bus and train network goes everywhere it is needed, everyone can afford it and it is fully accessible to people of all physical abilities. It is owned by the people, not private companies, so there is no profit motive. There is simply no reason to own a car; it wouldn't make economic sense. Especially as you could hire or share an electric one for occasional use.

'A mere utopia!' I hear you cry.

'You may say I'm a dreamer…' But wait. I lived, for a few years, in a city where the buses were indeed so cheap and reliable that virtually no-one needed to own a car. No, not Oslo, not Stockholm, and certainly not Utopia. Sheffield, UK. Or, as it was jokingly known in the 1980s, the Socialist Republic of South Yorkshire. I knew people of all ages and income brackets: everyone walked, cycled or took the bus. And because it wasn't worth owning a car, there were so few cars on the roads that cycling felt really safe, even on those steep hills. At the end of the 1980s, I moved away from Sheffield and stopped cycling – because there were so many more cars on the roads. (Today, sadly, Sheffield's streets are as clogged and smelly and toxic as any in the UK.)

Electric vehicles (EVs), I learn from transport expert David Janner-Klausner, PhD, are actually more efficient (use less electricity) when stopping and starting. This is why electric hail-and-ride buses, delivery lorries and garbage trucks work well. However, electric vehicles, he adds, produce just as much pollution from tyre dust as ordinary cars. David is a sustainable transport and planning specialist and co-founder of Commonplace, a leading UK platform for online consultation about the built environment and transport. We'll hear more from him shortly.

What are the obstacles to implementing such a vision? I'll start with what I regard as the most serious obstacle, and possibly the least known. EVs are non-polluting locally (in the place where they are driven). But their huge batteries rely on minerals such as lithium, nickel and cobalt, sourced from vulnerable parts of the planet. Three quarters of the world's lithium is concentrated in three Latin American countries: Argentina, Brazil and Chile, although lithium mining is beginning now in Cornwall, in South West England. At least half of all the world's cobalt is found in the Democratic Republic of the Congo, a country ravaged by war and extreme poverty. There is child labour in those cobalt mines. Neither the kids nor adults have protective gear. The cobalt is dug out with forced labour in unsafe, unregulated mines, as discovered and documented by Amnesty International, Unicef and The Borgen Project (www.borgenproject.org). These organisations are trying to do something about this but, as ever, are up against the greed of companies who will stop at nothing to make a fast buck.

Nickel, another metal that EV batteries need, is found in Indonesia, Australia and Brazil. One of the last surviving uncontacted tribes in Indonesia, the Hongana Manyawa, live in the rainforest of Halmahera Island, in tune with their ecosystem and doing no harm to anyone. Unfortunately for them, there are nickel deposits in the ground there and the excavators are already moving in, with the agreement of the Indonesian government.[37] The peoples' land, way of life and their very lives are endangered by nickel mining. Find out more from Survival International.

I'm so sorry to throw a spanner in the EV works. Nothing's simple, is it? Just when we thought we had a solution, somebody mentions the supply chain. Whoops.

I put this problem to Dr David Janner-Klausner, the transport expert. He feels we are in the early, 'goldrush' phase of such mining and that it will soon be put on a more ethical footing. I'm not so confident. What David also points out, however, is that EV batteries can be repurposed, reused and recycled, thus vastly reducing the amount of such batteries we need. He adds that as charging facilities improve, smaller batteries will become more acceptable, thus using fewer resources. It does come down to quantity – and thus to restraint. It seems to me that the only answer is to massively reduce private car ownership – of any kind of car – almost to zero, with the exceptions listed above. But this is where we come up against another major obstacle: the love affair.

Many people are deeply in love with their cars. They experience their cars as an extension of their home, even of their self. They just love the private space, their own choice of music, the sense of freedom. Perhaps this is how our ancestors felt two hundred years ago, riding a horse – except that their experience of freedom was real, because they didn't spend hours stuck in gridlock behind a queue of other horses! This attachment is not just about convenience, and it's a hard nut to crack. Some people don't want to be on a bus or train partly because they don't want to share space with strangers; so, if they do have to use public transport, they stick their earphones in and stare down at their phones. (Secret tip: if you get talking to other people, they cease to be strangers.)

But imagine if buses and trains were beautiful, spacious and comfortable, as well as clean, cheap and reliable. Dr David Janner-Klausner says that such trains do exist, in Finland – they even contain play areas for children, making long journeys with kids much less stressful! And if cars of all kinds were really expensive, priced as the luxury items they actually are? (If you think, by the way, that properly funded and fully nationalised/

locally owned public transport is a socialist concept, you'd be right; so is the National Health Service.)

Moving in the Right Direction

In my ecological medicine practice, when working with a sick person my golden rule has always been: 'Put the good stuff in before you take the bad stuff out.' Meaning, in the clinical context, add in all the missing nutrients, to optimum levels, before starting to remove the toxins. This makes the body strong enough to cope with the detox, but it is also the case that the nutrients themselves help to push the toxins out. I think the analogy here is fairly precise: we need to put in place affordable public transport that is really fabulous in every way, and then people will more easily let go of private car ownership – and the hassle of finding and paying for a parking place – for aesthetic, social, ecological and health reasons as well as economic reasons. Without coercion. Because coercion is never okay.

So, let's look briefly at some current attempts to improve urban air quality. Paris, under mayor Anne Hidalgo, has a bike-hire scheme, Vélib', with nearly 20,000 bikes; 60 per cent of them are old-fashioned mechanical bikes, 40 per cent electric. Each month in Paris there are nearly five million bicycle journeys. Until recently, Paris also had an electric car-sharing scheme, Autolib. Diesel vehicles and the most polluting petrol ones will be banned by 2025. And there is a tax on SUVs and heavy (non-electric) vehicles. The air is already improving; you can read more on the Paris schemes and much else about combatting air pollution in Tim Smedley's excellent book, *Clearing the Air*.[38]

Stockholm will ban all petrol and diesel cars from its city centre in December 2024, and in 2025 the area covered by the ban will expand. London, under mayor Sadiq Khan, has introduced an Ultra-Low Emission Zone, ULEZ, charging the most polluting vehicles a fee, but also giving out £160 million in a 'scrappage scheme' to anyone who wants to upgrade to a less polluting vehicle. (A congestion charge for any vehicle entering the city centre has been in place since 2003.) The London Air Quality Network (www.londonair.org.uk) is monitoring air quality in London and south-east England. There are comparable schemes to the ULEZ in Birmingham (see www.brumbreathes.co.uk), Bristol and Leeds.

Has the London ULEZ improved the air quality? The GLA says yes, absolutely. But so far, the answer from scientists seems to be: 'Um, well, maybe a bit'.[39] And how do the citizens feel about it? While some people react to the ULEZ by clamouring about the additional charge and the restriction on their freedom to drive, others, including myself, feel that it hasn't gone far enough. It's too timid. But as with all restrictions on car use, people will not be happy unless seriously good public transport has been put in place first, as envisaged above. And unless they feel they have been properly consulted.

Oxford is an interesting case; a city full of cyclists but with plenty of motorised transport too. I interviewed (by email) someone who is a resident of Oxford; not a transport expert at all, but a professional singer (so I guess he cares about his lungs even more than most of us do). He seems to me to present a balanced range of responses to Oxford's admittedly controversial Low Traffic Neighbourhoods (LTNs).[40] Here is what he says:

> There has been huge outcry about LTNs, including outrage at what some think is a corrupt council pushing through changes against the will of Oxford citizens, and doing sham consultations. There is so much 'noise' around this, it seems hard to make sense of it all.
>
> There is no doubt that the LTNs have led to certain roads on the outskirts of the city getting much more clogged at certain times of day. That is to be expected. I thought the whole point was to push traffic out of the centre and residential areas, and, in the long term, reduce people's car use and encourage them to find alternative methods of travel. I have friends who are part of local and national movements to create greener environments, safer streets, and more cycling and walking. I very much support them and their mission. Other friends have bewailed the LTNs and have nothing good to say about them, often merging the comments with conspiracy theories about the council, the government etc. The complaints seem to centre around traffic jams at key moments in the day when people want to get somewhere quickly (commuting and school runs), access for businesses (e.g. mobile repair services) and the vulnerable and immobile. I have been distressed to

> hear of nurses having to give up work, because longer journey times mean they cannot do the school run and get to their shift in time.
>
> My understanding is that emergency services are not damaged by the LTNs. I get the impression that the majority of complaints come down to 'This is really inconvenient for me, and I don't want to have to change any aspect of my previous lifestyle.' Personally, I think that generations after us, who will suffer far more than us from the legacy of our dependency on non-renewables, will wonder why on earth we didn't do anything to prevent the climate catastrophe. Yes, it's inconvenient, but I think it's worth it.
>
> But I would add that Oxford introduced these LTNs without enough supportive measures. For example, they could have improved the public transport infrastructure, and incentivised people to use it more. And they could instigate a system whereby certain number-plates could trigger a bollard to go down and let a vehicle through if it belonged to a vulnerable person, or a health worker (like the nurses I mentioned). I suppose there could be quite a few exceptions like that, and I think it's worth looking into. Yes, we need to make people change their car use, but that should not penalise people who already need the community's support for their lives to be viable and not a misery. Builders etc. now have to use longer routes to get from their suppliers to their clients – so charge them more and get less done. Of course, there are losses to the current 'smoothness' of life, but we all need to sacrifice current convenience for the future health of our descendants and the planet.

I put some of these points to transport consultant Dr David Janner-Klausner. In particular, the nurses' disrupted journeys. Apparently transport experts call this a 'chained journey' – in another example that David gives me, a mum has to take her child to school, call in at the chemist for Grandma's prescription, drop it off at Grandma's and then go on to work. This is very difficult to do by existing public transport options; it could take all day. So, my 'utopian' vision takes a knock here. But David and colleagues in his field are working on it; it is precisely the kind of thing they are good at grappling with. Find out more at www.commonplace.is/low-traffic-neighbourhood-report.

It does seem rather obvious, even to someone like me who is not a transport expert, that if you simply divert cars from route X to route Y you will make route X less polluted but route Y more polluted, and possibly gridlocked. That's fine if you live along route X, but not if you live along route Y, even if, as a pedestrian, you sensibly take minor roads and walk as far as possible from the kerb (this does actually make a difference to how much pollution you inhale.[41]) These schemes clearly have to become far more democratic, sophisticated, fully thought out and genuinely consulted-upon. But we do need way fewer cars overall, so, I come back to the need for superb, properly funded public transport. And bicycles.

Bicycles, David says, could be subsidised, so everyone could afford them. Lorries, he adds, are now being built with lower cabs, so the drivers can see cyclists better; that will keep them a lot safer. And the police need to be funded properly to prevent bicycle theft, which is rampant in many cities, including London. David points out that, if every online advert for a bike for sale had to include the bike's serial number, owners could spot who stole their bike and (if the police are functioning) get it back.

Anne Hidalgo, the mayor of Paris whose changes are cleaning up the city's air, was inspired by the work of the Franco-Columbian professor Carlos Moreno. It was Moreno who coined the term '15-minute cities', the idea being that everything you needed could be within a 15-minute walk, bike ride or bus ride from your home. 'Everything' includes school, work, shops, healthcare, leisure and entertainment. Sounds good to me, sounds like the reinvention of the village within the urban landscape. But it needs to be put in place first, properly, before we will be able to get people out of their cars once and for all and breathe freely again.

In conclusion, here's a story. I don't know with whom it originates, but I heard it in the early 1990s from Rabbi Zalman Schachter-Shalomi. It goes like this:

There is a big ship crossing the ocean. Many passengers, many cabins. One day, some passengers hear a strange banging sound coming from one of the cabins. Then the worrying sound of a pneumatic drill.

They call out to whoever is inside the cabin, 'Hey, what are you doing?' but there is no reply.

They go to fetch the captain. He too calls out, 'Hey, what do you think you are doing in there?' Again, initially, no reply. He asks again.

Eventually, the occupant of the cabin shouts, irritably, 'What does it sound like? I'm drilling a hole in the floor.'

'You are doing what?' cries the captain, aghast. 'You can't do that! If you make a hole in the floor, we'll all drown!'

'Oh, really?' replies the occupant. 'Well, sorry mate, I've paid for this cabin. It's my cabin, nothing to do with you. I can do exactly what I like in here.'

'But we'll drown!' repeat the captain and the passengers.

'Not my problem,' replies the occupant who has paid for his very own cabin.

Your freedom to drive your very own car, my freedom to breathe our shared air. In the end, we're all in the same boat.

CHAPTER FIVE

FIRE I: POISONOUS LIGHT

If only I had known, I should have become a watchmaker.

Attributed to Albert Einstein

This chapter, and the following one, are about the effects on our bodies of pollution that is physical rather than chemical. Physical pollution comes in the form of wavelengths of energy, rather than atoms and molecules of chemical 'stuff'. Einstein's equation ($E = mc^2$) tells us that energy and matter are 'ultimately' interchangeable; but we don't have to worry about 'ultimately' because we're discussing ordinary life on earth. However, here's another hard thing to get our heads around in physics: light is a form of electromagnetic energy. And all light can be conceived of as photons – discrete 'particles' of light – or as waves. It can behave as either, depending mostly on how physicists observe it.

The Electromagnetic Spectrum

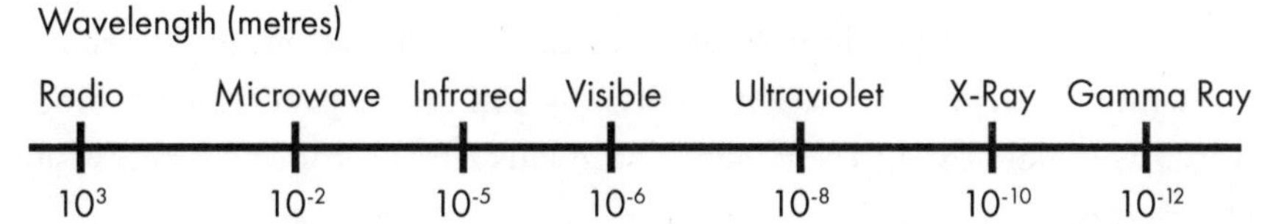

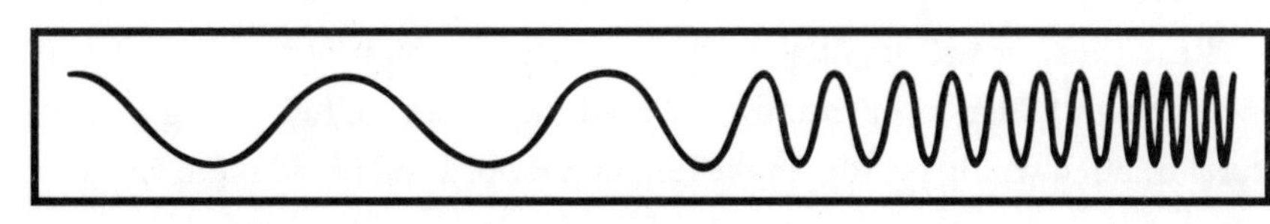

The diagram above shows the electromagnetic spectrum, the full range of all forms of radiation, or radiant energy. In the middle is the rainbow, the familiar spectrum of visible light. Red, orange, yellow, green, blue, indigo, violet (mnemonic: Richard Of York Gave Battle In Vain). The rest of the spectrum is invisible to us humans. Next door to the purple part of the visible spectrum is ultraviolet light; it has great cleansing and anti-microbial properties, and we need some of it to make vitamin D in our skin. But not too much, and not on its own; only naturally, as part of sunshine, so we'll be getting the healing rays of infrared light at the same time. Infrared light lies on the other side of the visible spectrum, next door to red light, and is calming, healing, warming and necessary to life. We humans give off infrared radiation from our bodies; that's one of the reasons it feels so good to hug someone.

We've evolved over millions of years with this narrow, middle section of the spectrum; just visible light, ultraviolet and infrared. Either side of this section are forms of electromagnetic (EM) energy that are alien to our bodies. They do exist way out in space, but until the past hundred or so years we haven't encountered them too much down here on earth (this is a controversial statement and I'll explain more later).

I've divided this subject into two chapters. In this chapter I'll deal with the various types of short-wavelength radiation – where they come from and what they do to us. This is the high frequency side of the spectrum: X-rays and gamma rays; also, alpha and beta radiation. Gamma rays have even shorter wavelengths and higher frequencies than X-rays.

Nuclear Radiation

It is 1980 and I'm on the wards in St James's Hospital (locally known as Jimmy's), Leeds, UK. I'm a fourth-year medical student and this is part of our three-month paediatric rotation. Right now, I'm on the paediatric oncology ward, where almost all the children have leukaemia – cancer of the white blood cells.

'Read these notes,' says the professor, unceremoniously pushing a pile of thick, brown folders over to me, 'and read them thoroughly.' Being a rather literal-minded young person, I take him at his word and I read them all, cover to cover, including their front pages. The front page has details like name, address, date of birth and father's occupation. Something strikes me immediately. The addresses – they're all in or very close to the village of Seascale, in Cumbria. Postcode CA20. Next to the Windscale (later Sellafield) nuclear reactor. That's quite a long way from Leeds. I see that these children have been sent over the Pennines from a hospital in Carlisle; I guess they don't have the facilities there to do chemotherapy for children. Then I notice something else: father's occupation. Most of the dads of these very sick children are working at the Windscale nuclear reactor. A chill runs down my spine.

'Sir,' I ask the professor when I get a chance, 'all the patients here are from near the Windscale nuclear power plant. And most of their fathers work there. Have these children got some kind of radiation sickness?'

'Miss Goodman,' comes the stern reply, 'I am a clinician. My job is to treat my patients. I do not enquire about causes; I leave that to the epidemiologists.'

Epidemiologists are doctors or scientists, usually with a master's degree in public health, who study statistical trends in illnesses. They look for patterns, like clusters of illness in particular places or at particular moments in time. So, forty-four years on from that encounter on the wards of Jimmy's, we'll have a look at what they've found, including the significant clusters of leukaemia and other cancers, especially among children, around Sellafield[1] and other nuclear power plants.[2] (There was a huge public outcry about the leukaemia cases around Windscale, and the main response of the owners, British Nuclear Fuels Limited (BNFL), was to change Windscale's name to Sellafield in 1981.)

But first, we need to discuss what nuclear radiation is, where it comes from, how it gets into us and what it does to our bodies. Then we'll clear up a few important misunderstandings with crucial health implications and swiftly survey the history of nuclear radiation leaks and accidents and the resulting huge excesses of illness. And we'll venture briefly into how the dangers of nuclear radiation were (and still are) denied, the leaks and accidents covered up and the truthful scientists sacked. Sorry, it's politics again. Lastly, we'll see what we can do to protect ourselves; there are a couple of really simple things. But we can only protect ourselves from a danger if we know we're being exposed to it.

First, a word about terminology. Many of the books and papers on this subject use the phrase 'low-level radiation'. But 'low level' is a misnomer. In fact, the biological effects of so-called 'low-level' radiation are devastating and long-lasting; 'low level' does not mean 'low impact on our health'. We'll see later how this misnaming came about.

What Is Nuclear Radiation?

We have to do just a little bit of chemistry and physics here. Bear with me; it'll be worth it to understand this.

Everything on earth is composed of atoms and there are about one hundred different types, each constituting a particular element. Carbon, oxygen, nitrogen, hydrogen, iodine, iron, sodium, calcium, zinc and sulphur are examples of elements. You can see all one hundred plus of them if you look up the periodic table of the elements. Each atom is in turn composed of three types of subatomic particle: protons, neutrons and electrons. The nucleus, or centre of the atom, is made of protons and neutrons. A proton is positively charged and a neutron has no charge; as its name suggests, it's electrically neutral. Protons and neutrons have about the same mass as each other. Electrons, by contrast, are about two thousand times smaller/lighter than a proton or neutron, and carry a negative electric charge equal and opposite to the proton's charge. The electrons whizz around the nucleus at top speed and at a relatively vast distance from it. The atom is mostly empty space. Think miniature solar system, with the sun as the nucleus and the planets as the electrons. That's not precise, but it'll do.

Each atom has an atomic number, which is its number of protons, and also an atomic mass, which is its protons + neutrons. Normally, an atom is electrically neutral, because its electrons balance out its protons. Electrons get to be exchanged or shared when atoms of different elements combine to form compound substances, but the resulting substance is still electrically neutral overall. So much for the chemistry; now here comes the physics.

When we split the atom, whether to make weapons of war or for nuclear energy production, we mess with this fundamental structure of matter. Nuclear fission does what it says on the tin; it splits the nucleus of the atom. This results in loose neutrons flying around wildly and in 'unstable isotopes'. An isotope is a variant of an atom; it has the usual number of protons and electrons, but a different number of neutrons. Some isotopes occur in nature; atoms with a different-from-usual number of neutrons. But these natural isotopes tend, on the whole, to be stable; they don't go in for radioactive decay. The isotopes produced by nuclear fission, however, are unstable; they 'decay' into other isotopes and eventually into other elements – this is the alchemist's dream turned nightmare – and in the process they release a lethal package of energy in the form of alpha, beta or gamma radiation. The radiation produced, whether alpha, beta or gamma, is known as ionising radiation. It displaces electrons from atoms in living tissue, thus breaking the chemical bonds that hold one atom to another in our bodies. So, we become 'ionised', electrically charged, in an unnatural way. This is extremely risky, especially to our DNA; more on this shortly.

Alpha, beta and gamma radiation are not the same. Alpha 'rays' are not rays at all; they are actually alpha particles, consisting of two protons and two neutrons stuck together, without any electrons, and travel extremely fast. They are emitted by radioisotopes, such as uranium and plutonium, and pack a huge punch of energy. They don't penetrate very far, but any cells in their path will be seriously damaged or destroyed.[3] Beta 'rays' or rather beta particles are high-speed electrons, which penetrate about a centimetre into us and cause ionisation damage en route. They can't get through clothing, but don't be falsely reassured by that; clothing doesn't protect you from particles emitting beta rays (or any other radiation) from inside your body, which is what happens when we inhale or ingest radioactive particles. Gamma rays, also produced by radioactive decay, can pass through steel and concrete and do tremendous damage to living tissue, including causing cancer.

Nearly done with the physics. Radioactive isotopes (which are also known as radioisotopes, radionuclides or radioactive nuclides – just in case you wanted a bit more terminology!) each decay at different rates; their 'half-life' is how long it takes for half the radiation they emit to be emitted and gone. For radioactive iodine (I-131) this is eight days. Please note, this does NOT mean it will all be gone in sixteen days; it means that half is gone in eight days, then half the REMAINDER in another eight, and so on. (In other words, radioactive substances decay exponentially. Mathematically, the radiation emitted will never quite reach zero.) So radioactive iodine, released from nuclear accidents and nuclear weapons testing, is a major danger in the first few weeks after an accident or explosion. It's a danger particularly to our thyroid glands and especially to the very young, including the foetus. We can protect ourselves against this by having jolly good levels of safe, ordinary, non-radioactive iodine in our bodies to start off with (see *SAITT*, pages 75–76).

For strontium-90 (^{90}SR or Sr-90), the half-life is twenty-nine years, which gives it plenty of time to keep emitting radiation and irradiating us from within if it gets into our bones, as it does after nuclear releases. We'll see shortly why strontium heads for the bone just as iodine heads for the thyroid gland, and how we can, to some extent, protect ourselves against it. Caesium-137 (Cs-137), another important radioisotope, has a half-life of thirty years. The half-life of naturally occurring uranium, U-238, is 4.5 billion years – it's as old as the earth. We wouldn't need to worry about uranium if it had been left in the ground, but it's been mined, and used in nuclear power stations and weapons, for some decades now. Uranium used as fuel in nuclear reactors turns into plutonium (Pu), a totally human-made element. Pu-240 has a half-life of about 6,560 years, and Pu-239 of more than 24,000 years. This is why nuclear sites remain radioactive and dangerous for many, many generations.

Where Does Nuclear Radiation Come From?

Firstly, it comes from nuclear explosions, both intentional and accidental. Nuclear weapons testing began in the 1940s (check out the film *Oppenheimer*) and two atomic bombs were deliberately dropped on Hiroshima and Nagasaki in Japan in 1945. Nuclear testing then continued intensively until 1963, when a treaty between the US and USSR banned atmospheric and on-the-ground testing. But it didn't ban underground testing, which continued, especially by France and China, until the Comprehensive Test Ban Treaty of 1996. Even after this, India, Pakistan and North Korea have sporadically continued with 'testing', the most recent test (at time of writing) being in 2017.

Secondly, nuclear radiation comes from accidents at nuclear reactor sites like those at Windscale (1957), Kyshtym (also 1957), Three Mile Island (1979), Chernobyl (1986) and Fukushima (2011) and many more, some of which we haven't heard much about. Thirdly, it comes from 'licensed releases': permitted, perfectly legal, regular leaks of radioactive material into the sea and the atmosphere.

Fourthly, ionising radiation also comes from X-ray machines, which have been used diagnostically in medicine for a long time. X-rays are different from alpha, beta and gamma radiation in that their source is almost always external; the X-ray machine is outside you and it is perfectly possible to shield the parts of your body that are not being X-rayed from the radiation. This means asking the radiographer for a lead apron; in my experience most hospitals still have them, but staff are sometimes reluctant to go along the corridor and fetch one for you; they're very heavy to carry! They will argue that: 'The doses these days are too low to worry about' – but I'm not convinced. If I ever need an X-ray, I insist on a lead apron, however long it takes them to find one. And, of course, the potential damage from X-rays depends on how many you have – the gene-damaging effects are cumulative – and on how old you are; the younger you are, the more hazardous X-rays become. As with any radiation, the foetus is the most vulnerable of all.

X-raying the foetus in the womb is something that is, mercifully, never done today, thanks to a pioneering doctor called Alice Stewart, who worked in preventive medicine at Oxford. Her goddaughter had died of leukaemia at age three; leukaemia was rare, then, in the early 1950s, but Alice suspected (rightly) that it was on the increase. Her study, published in the *British Medical Journal* in 1958, confirmed her suspicion that obstetric X-rays had something to do with the increase.[4] She found that the chance of having been X-rayed *in utero* (in the womb) was significantly higher for those children who died of leukaemia than for those who were alive and well.

Neither the medical establishment nor the burgeoning nuclear industry were at all happy with Dr Stewart's results and of course tried to discredit her. But four years later another study, this time in America, confirmed what she had found; cancer mortality (for leukaemia and all other childhood cancers) was 40 per cent higher in children who had been X-rayed before birth than in those who had not.[5] You would think, given these results, that the X-raying of pregnant women would have stopped there and then, in 1962. But no; for reasons of inertia as well as vested interests, scientific discoveries are often very, very slow to percolate down into clinical practice. Babies in the womb continued to be X-rayed right up until the 1970s and even the beginning of the 1980s in the UK. X-rays, however, are not the only reason for the increase in childhood cancer, as we'll see. If you want to find out more about the brave and amazing Dr Alice Stewart, check out this biography by Professor Gayle Greene: *The Woman Who Knew Too Much: Alice Stewart and the Secrets of Radiation*.

How Does Nuclear Radiation Get into Our Bodies?

Fallout from nuclear establishments gets into the air, the rain and the soil. Children playing on the beach at Seascale may be inhaling radioactive dust; the particles are tiny enough to get not just into the lungs but through the walls of the alveoli (air sacs) and into the circulation, thus to all the cells and organs of the body. Then it rains. Whatever radioactive particles are suspended in the air will be washed into the rivers and the soil and, once in the soil, they will be absorbed by plants. So, strontium-90 and iodine-131 and similar radionuclides get taken up into the grass, which is then eaten by sheep and cows. Thus, these radioactive isotopes get concentrated up the food chain, so both milk and meat become contaminated.

After the disaster at Chernobyl (where the fire burnt for at least ten days), the winds blew the radioactive cloud all around the globe and mortality rates shot up everywhere.[6] Studies in the US linked the increase in radioactive iodine in milk directly to the increase in deaths.[7] They also linked the rise in the strontium-90 content of milk to the increase in infant mortality; one of the many other times this happened was after a series of accidents at the Savannah River nuclear plant in South Carolina operated by Du Pont,[8] whom we came across in chapter 3. These accidents, culminating in 1970, were kept secret for decades.[9] Infant mortality in South Carolina increased massively in an era (the early 1970s) when it was actually falling across the rest of the US. Strontium-90 got into fish as well as milk, and the people, unknowing, ate the fish.[10] Cancer rates went up accordingly, especially bone cancer and leukaemia. Myeloid leukaemia is effectively a cancer of the bone marrow, which is where many of our white blood cells are made; if there is Sr-90 in the bone, the marrow is being continually irradiated from within.[11]

Shortly after the Savannah River accidents, the level of Sr-90 in human bones in the region was found to be the highest ever recorded. The US government's response to this finding was to decide to stop measuring the level of Sr-90 in bones![12] Strontium-90 in the bones of a pregnant woman will leach out into her bloodstream and go through the umbilical cord into her placenta and her baby, which is one of the reasons that miscarriages, stillbirths and infant mortality (deaths in the first year of life) go up so high in the months and years after these disasters.

Why does Sr-90, whether from meat, milk, fish or even plant food, go into bones in the first place? It's because Sr-90 looks to the body like calcium; it is in the same chemical group, group 2, of the periodic table of the elements (so is radium). The body is expecting calcium and mistakes Sr-90 for it, so Sr-90 becomes incorporated into bone structure. Now, a tiny amount of non-radioactive strontium is a normal component of bone. But the body bases its decisions about which substance goes where on chemistry, not physics; it recognises the outer electron structure of an atom, not its nucleus, so it cannot differentiate radioactive from non-radioactive strontium. In just the same way, the thyroid gland cannot differentiate between radioactive and non-radioactive iodine; it's only the nucleus of the atom that's different, and the body doesn't 'see' that, it only 'sees' the electrons orbiting around. This is a major reason why our bodies have virtually no defence against radioactive substances.

Radioactivity doesn't stay in the area where it's released. Wind and rain, rivers and oceans carry it everywhere, so the level of risk to any one person depends not only on how near they live to the nuclear accident or deliberate (permitted) nuclear leak, but equally on whether they are downwind of it, and also on the level of rainfall in the area where they live. After the Chernobyl disaster, Wales was the worst affected part of Britain, because it has the highest rainfall.[13] And Wales also had its own nuclear power station, Trawsfynydd, now mercifully closed down due to public campaigning by the Low Level Radiation Campaign, although I believe there are moves afoot to reopen it. Cancer rates among people living within 3.5 km of Trawsfynydd, or downwind of it, were found to be significantly higher than those in the rest of Wales and England.[14]

All this came on top of radioactive discharges reaching the north Wales coast from Sellafield in Cumbria, via the Irish Sea. Radioactive particles in the smoke from the Windscale fire also reached the east coast of Ireland, where Dr Patricia Sheehan recorded an unusual cluster of babies born with a chromosomal disorder, Trisomy 21, or Down's Syndrome, in 1983.[15] Dr Sheehan became a determined campaigner against nuclear power, but unfortunately died in a car accident in 1994. Many nuclear power plants are sited on the coast, including Sellafield (Windscale) and Diablo Canyon; they discharge their radioactive waste directly into the sea, where winds blow it back onto the land as particles that we can inhale.[16] And, once in the sea, it gets into the fish.

Scotland, like Wales, gets a lot of rain. Both Wales and Scotland saw a sharp increase in cases of infant leukaemia in the two years following the Chernobyl accident, as did other countries in Europe. These children could have been affected while in the womb or even before, by the effects of the fallout on the egg and sperm of their parents. These increases occurred despite the confident predictions of the UK National Radiological Protection Board that there would be no increase.[17]

Accidents do happen. When the nuclear facility at Windscale caught fire in 1957, radioactive smoke was blown all over Britain and northern Europe.[18] It contained and distributed many types of radioactive particles, including iodine-131, which, as above, contaminated the milk. Millions of litres of milk had to be discarded because of the immense risk to the human thyroid gland.[19] But even before (and after) the fire, there were countless unrecorded releases of 'thousands of millions of highly radioactive particles ... found in gardens and homes, including the larders in Seascale'.[20] It's still going on – and is perfectly legal.

Biological Effects: What Does Nuclear Radiation Do to Our Bodies?

Nuclear radiation is ionising radiation, so it produces 'free radicals', electrically charged particles that damage all our cell structures, especially our cell membranes[21] and our genes. The body has some mechanisms to deal with free radicals, including the enzyme superoxide dismutase, but these defences evolved to deal only with the small amount of free radicals produced momentarily by our normal mitochondrial metabolism; they quickly get overwhelmed by nuclear radiation. And excesses of free radicals are associated with almost all known diseases.

We have seen that the radioactive fission product Sr-90 heads for the bones and teeth[22] (so does radium) and it is strongly implicated in bone cancer[23] as well as in leukaemia, but it also seems to be implicated in often-fatal congenital heart disease in babies.[24] And it can cause this at levels well below the so-called background radiation levels; 'natural background radiation' is a misleading and irrelevant comparison when discussing human-made fission products like Sr-90 and I-131. We evolved on this planet over millions of years with natural background radiation, such as that given off by granite rocks or reaching us from the outer cosmos (albeit filtered through the atmosphere). But both Sr-90 and I-131 form part of the fallout from nuclear accidents, along with caesium, uranium, plutonium and several others.

Radioactive iodine, I-131, released after the Chernobyl fire, the Fukushima disaster and many similar events, has led to a significant increase in cancer of the thyroid gland. Greenpeace's study done in 2016[25] showed a nearly tenfold increase in thyroid cancer among children exposed to the radioactive fallout in Ukraine (Chernobyl is in Ukraine). In a part of Belarus close to Chernobyl, there were babies born with thyroid cancer.[26] And we've seen similar effects in Fukushima in Japan.[27] Thyroid cancer is normally an extremely rare disease in children. So how does this occur?

The thyroid gland needs iodine to make thyroid hormone (thyroxine), so will absorb it eagerly from the bloodstream. As described above in relation to strontium, the body can't distinguish between normal (essential) iodine and radioactive (toxic) iodine, because the difference is in the nucleus of the atom, not in the electrons, so the body can't 'see' the difference. Once radioactive iodine gets into the thyroid gland (or any body part; most of our other organs need some iodine too), it irradiates the tissue from within. This is not like a one-off blast from an X-ray machine; it's chronic, internal, ongoing.

A thyroid gland already full up with normal, non-radioactive iodine is better protected. But do you need to protect yourself? Apart from the fact that, even in the absence of radioactive fallout, the thyroid gland needs plenty of iodine to be healthy, are you worried that you might be living in the vicinity of a nuclear power plant? Look up 'UK map of nuclear power stations', or the US equivalent, and find out. There are quite a lot of them about; you may be nearer than you think. And now we come to the crux of this troubling issue.

Nuclear radiation damages the DNA in our cells: our genes.[28] DNA (deoxyribonucleic acid) is a complex and sophisticated set of molecular instructions for the formation of a living being. It tells the body which proteins to manufacture (we are made of proteins), which biochemical processes to turn on or off, and when – and more. Think of DNA as the script of a play. If the actors are reading the correct play, it will manifest as *Hamlet*. But if the script has been tampered with, whole passages deleted and replaced with nonsense, it won't be *Hamlet*. It won't hang together and it won't make sense, still less be moving and profound. It will be a mess.

That is the best analogy I can come up with for what DNA is and for what radiation does to it. The resultant distortions in the genetic script are called mutations. Mutations eventually cause cancer in the person or animal in whom they occur. Leukaemia appears quite soon after exposure, because it is a cancer of cells that multiply very rapidly. Solid cancers take longer to appear; the lag time in adults is often measured in decades. But something else can happen before cancer appears; because the radiation-induced mutations are now part of the person's genetic material, they are in the egg or sperm. They get transmitted to future generations. There are several animal studies showing this,[29] and also studies of the families of 'nuclear veterans', men who worked in the nuclear atmospheric testing programmes, so were substantially exposed to nuclear radiation. These studies have shown increases in congenital illnesses, miscarriages, stillbirths and infant deaths among their children and their grandchildren.[30]

Uranium. If we are talking about genetic damage, we need to talk about uranium. It's the commonest component of nuclear fallout because it's the main ingredient in nuclear power production, nuclear weapons manufacture and nuclear waste processing. It is not only radioactive, it is one of the 'DNA-seeking' isotopes. It is attracted to our DNA.[31] Chemically, although it is not exactly in the same group as calcium and strontium (both of which bind strongly to DNA), uranium does resemble them in having the same number of electrons (two) in its outermost orbit. Normally, there is a lot of calcium closely associated with our DNA. Uranium, it seems, can displace it. Here, the problem is not so much radiation given out directly by the decay of uranium atoms, but the fact that they absorb 447 times more photon energy from natural background radiation than calcium would.[32] And then they re-emit this radiation – directly into our DNA. It seems that the effects of this, in terms of genetic damage, have been underestimated at least 1,000-fold.[33] Shortly, we'll see why.

Uranium weapons have been used in conflicts since the first Gulf War in 1991. As I write, they are being employed in the war in Ukraine. It turns out that this has significantly raised the amount of uranium in the UK, according to measurements recorded at the Atomic Weapons Establishment in Aldermaston, Berkshire, England.[34] These tiny, insoluble nanoparticles of radioactive uranium oxide are travelling west on the wind, as did the fallout from Chernobyl – and we inhale them[35] – and they remain in the environment for an indefinite period of time. As if we needed another reason to try to bring an end to war.

Insoluble uranium oxide particles have been found on the coasts near at least three UK nuclear power stations: Sellafield in Cumbria, north-west England, Dounreay in Scotland and Hinkley Point near the Severn Estuary in Somerset, south-west England. Tidal action breaks these up into smaller and smaller particles, and the smaller they become the more dangerous they are to us because the alpha rays they emit can penetrate further into us (whereas in bigger particles, the particle itself absorbs some of its alpha emissions).[36] But doesn't the Environment Agency keep an eye on this? No. It doesn't monitor uranium. And Geiger counters don't pick up alpha-emitters.[37] Similarly, UNSCEAR 2000 (UN Committee on the Effects of Atomic Radiation) looked at licensed releases from every operating nuclear reactor in the world between 1990 and 1997 (there hasn't been such a survey since). And yet the UNSCEAR report didn't include uranium (or the still-radioactive thorium into which it decays).[38] Go figure.

There is a triple whammy here. Radiation causes mutations, which eventually lead to cancer, but it also damages the cells of the immune system whose job is to spot cancerous cells and destroy them before they can multiply and form a tumour. And radiation, in damaging our genes, will inevitably damage some of those genes whose task is specifically to suppress cancer; they are called 'tumour-suppressor genes' and will get zapped by radiation along with many other genes. All this, along with the toxic, carcinogenic chemicals we've discussed in the previous four chapters, is undoubtedly responsible for the massive increase in cancer we've seen over the past century, from a rare disease to something that now one in two of us will suffer from. (And despite what we're told, the increase is nothing to do with ageing, as explained in my first book, *SAITT*, on pages 231–233. Cancer rates are rising fastest among the young.)

Children are the most vulnerable to all these effects, the foetus the most vulnerable of all. The younger you are, the faster you are growing. And the smaller you are, the higher your surface-area-to-volume ratio (a greater proportion of your body is surface) and therefore the greater your capacity to absorb all kinds of pollution from your environment. Dr Alice Stewart showed back in the 1950s that the radiation dose considered safe for an adult is vastly more dangerous for a baby in the womb,[39] and today, preconception damage is a very real risk in our nuclear-powered world.[40] Until the 1980s there was no such thing as a children's hospice. Now, there's a charity shop raising funds for one on many a high street.

Crucial Misunderstandings, Dangerous Fallacies

A lot of confusion has been created around how much radiation exposure, if any, is safe. Spoiler alert: my belief is that there is no safe dose, especially for the young. But what confusion? How has it arisen? And what consequences has it had?

It goes back to the bombs that were dropped on Hiroshima and Nagasaki in 1945. After the bombings, it seems the American government suddenly discovered a guilty conscience and set up a long-running study to examine the effects on the health of those who survived the blasts. But this 'life-span study' (LSS), which is still used as a basis by many scientists today, only looks at the effects of external radiation, which the survivors were exposed to at the moment of the explosion. It takes no account of the ongoing internal radiation to which the people would have been subjected over the ensuing years, by inhaling radioactive particles of uranium, plutonium and so on in the fallout, and also by swallowing them in food as they became incorporated into soil, plants and animals, as described above.

Therefore, the LSS did not find much more cancer in those who had been relatively near the explosion (near enough to feel the heat but far enough away to survive) compared to those who had been a bit further away at the time. This is because those who were further away, it turns out, were equally exposed to the radioactive fallout as it was spread by the wind and rain over the years. And that was the major factor. When a proper comparison was finally done of all those people, by a Japanese scientist, it turned out that all the survivors in the general vicinity had at least a three-fold increase in cancer deaths when compared with those in a genuine control group, living much further away.[41] The LSS ignored the effects of the 'Black Rain' that fell in that part of Japan, black because it was contaminated with tiny particles of uranium-234.[42] So, the precedent was set, over seventy years ago, when measuring how much radiation a person had been exposed to, to consider only the external dose and to ignore internal contamination, even though the latter is ongoing, not momentary, and far more important.

A related problem arose at the same time, about the 'absorbed dose' of radiation. Nuclear radiation releases energy. But the current model of calculating how much energy is released into a human body by irradiation makes a big and erroneous assumption; it assumes that the energy is evenly distributed over the person's whole body. This may be true if you go for an X-ray, but, if you have inhaled or ingested some radioactive particles, then the radiation is not at all evenly distributed. Those particles will be in a particular location in your body, according to where their chemistry takes them. Most likely sitting on your DNA, in fact.[43] So what matters is how much radiation is reaching your genes. One mutated cell can lead to many mutated 'daughter' cells, and eventually to cancer. So, a level of radiation that might indeed be virtually harmless if it were spread out evenly over your entire body is in fact very rarely spread out like that. The 'radiation density' or dose in a particular cell in your body can be huge. And it only takes one cell…

Richard Bramhall of the Low Level Radiation Campaign told me of Professor Chris Busby's brilliant analogy to help us understand this. Professor Busby says: 'It's an averaging error, like believing it makes no difference whether you sit by the fire to warm yourself or eat a burning coal.'[44] The point being that, whatever the overall amount of heat/energy, what matters is how it is concentrated in one particular part – or cell, or molecule – within the body. But how could such fundamental errors have remained unchanged and unchallenged for so many decades?

They haven't actually remained unchallenged, but the scientists who have pointed out the errors – and the resultant vast underestimation of the damage being caused to our health – have mostly been silenced, sacked and ridiculed. For the simple reason that nuclear power is Very Big Money, and if it were to be publicly acknowledged that what the nuclear industry calls a 'low dose' is in fact a potentially lethal dose for your cells, your genes – well, their vast profits would be threatened. 'Twas ever thus, it seems. Tobacco, asbestos – it's the same story. The industry pays its own scientists to rubbish the results they don't like. Truly independent funding for serious research is hard to come by. Meanwhile, governments and companies keep building nuclear power stations, and the cancer rates keep going up. Especially among children.

The model of risk that the nuclear industry uses is intended to reassure us, so we don't get active and threaten their profits. But it's a false reassurance; the model has clearly and conclusively been shown to be wrong, time and time again, and most recently by Professor Busby's brilliant and comprehensive 2022 paper, 'Ionizing Radiation and Cancer: The Failure of the Risk Model'.[45]

Another deliberate misunderstanding on the part of the nuclear industry is to repeatedly claim, when faced with evidence such as the leukaemia clusters around Sellafield: 'But that amount of radiation can't possibly be the cause; it's no higher than natural background radiation.' This is disingenuous. We are clearly adapted to deal with natural background radiation; if it was as carcinogenic as the synthetic fission-products of the nuclear industry, the human race would never have survived. In fact, as Professor Busby points out,[46] there is experimental proof that exposure to human-made radiation causes different and far worse health effects than does natural background radiation.

The story of nuclear power and its hazards is a story of sickness, death, denial, cover-up and corruption. Even the pleas and warnings of eminent, Nobel-prize-winning scientists like Linus Pauling and Andrei Sakharov fell on deaf ears. Indeed, some of the scientists who had worked on the original nuclear bomb repented of their actions when they realised what the fallout was doing to people's bodies, and urged an end to the nuclear power and weapons programmes. They were ignored, marginalised or fired. It is estimated that, in the seventeen years from 1945 to 1962, 'the super-powers subjected the populations of the world to the fallout equivalent of 40,000 Hiroshima bombs.'[47] But this is not all in the past; new nuclear reactors continue to be built, to leak radioactive fallout and periodically to explode in catastrophic fires.

As I write, in December 2023, both the *Guardian* and the BBC are reporting worrying problems at Sellafield, now officially a nuclear decommissioning facility and 'widely regarded as the most hazardous nuclear site in the world.' Apparently, its computer systems have been cyber-attacked by hackers linked with Russia and China, and this has been going on since 2015 but senior staff have been covering up the security failures, and the 'Office for Nuclear Regulation' (ONR) has only just got on the case, so is busy covering up its own dereliction of duty as well as finally putting Sellafield into 'special measures', like a failing school.

The 'malware' affecting Sellafield's servers may compromise activities like moving nuclear waste, of which there are huge amounts. Sellafield contains 140 tonnes of plutonium, a legacy from the Cold War; the largest such store on the planet. It has also taken in radioactive waste from Sweden, Italy and other countries. Radioactive sludge is stored in a vast open-air pond that has a number of cracks in its concrete bottom and contaminated water has been leaking into the ground for several years. But the leak is apparently too deep to be accessible to repairs. Sellafield's CEO, Mr Hutton, therefore proposes to 'take the waste away for storage elsewhere'. But as we know, there is no 'away', there is no 'elsewhere'.

As well as nuclear waste, also stored at Sellafield and potentially accessible to hackers are 'disaster manuals', plans for what to do in case of an emergency like a foreign attack or indeed a nuclear disaster in Cumbria. Someone will always be half-asleep on duty; accidents happen.

And so, to the future.

What Shall We Do?

Small things and big things. The small things are: ensuring your own body has a good level of iodine to protect your thyroid gland from radioactive iodine. Make sure you have plenty of calcium and magnesium to protect your bones – and hence your bone marrow, where your white blood cells are made – from radioactive strontium. More on iodine, calcium and magnesium, from both food and supplements, in *SAITT*. Should you take a supplement of (non-radioactive) strontium itself? Well, opinion is divided, but I would say probably, just a little, occasionally. Especially if you have osteoporosis or are nursing a broken bone; some people find it speeds up bone healing. Clearly, safe strontium will go some way to keeping out radioactive strontium. But don't overdo it, and preferably do it in consultation with a nutritional practitioner. Strontium is supposed to be only a minor component of our bones.

The big things are these: inform yourself, think global and act local. In the UK, the Low Level Radiation Campaign (www.llrc.org) needs your support. But don't be misled by the phrase 'Low Level'. It's referring to what the nuclear industry calls 'low level', but, as we've seen, this so-called low level is catastrophic for our bodies; it was 'very low dose' exposure that caused so much leukaemia in babies all over Europe after the Chernobyl disaster.[48]

The charity Children with Cancer UK has commissioned the Low Level Radiation Campaign, headed by the devoted and hardworking Richard Bramhall, to produce a report, along with Peter Wilkinson, co-founder of Greenpeace, called 'Radiation and Reason: The Impact of Science on a Culture of Confusion'. I've read the first version; it is excellent. A second and final version should be out by the time this book is in your hands; it is intended for the general public and will be well worth reading.

Richard says the most effective action is to join a local campaign; check out the nuclear power station nearest you and see if there is a campaign to close it down. In Somerset there is www.stophinkley.org, which is trying, among other projects, to prevent EDF (Électricité de France) from dumping radioactive mud from the Severn Estuary right next door to Cardiff. Yes, that's what EDF plan to do. The people living near to and downwind of Hinkley Point power station have already been shown to have an excess of infant mortality and breast cancer.[49] EDF's plan would only extend those problems from north Somerset into south Wales.

Sometimes you may read that your local power station is being decommissioned – but keep an eye on it. Trawsfynydd in north Wales was closed down years ago due to a brilliant local campaign by WANA (Wales Anti-Nuclear Alliance), LLRC (Low Level Radiation Campaign) and others, but the nuclear authorities may be trying to rebuild it now.

We need to be campaigning for three things:

- For the nuclear industry and governments to start telling the truth about the health hazards of their very profitable, toxic fission products. Or at least to stop defunding and silencing the brave scientists who have been telling that truth all along.
- For all existing nuclear facilities to be closed down and safely decommissioned and, along with all locations where nuclear waste is dumped, to have permanent barriers erected around them, not holiday homes or housing estates built on them. They will be dangerous for thousands of years to come and need to stand only as a memorial to our folly. (A lot has been dumped into the sea. You can't build a barrier around the sea. But we could at least stop dumping radioactive waste into it).
- For no further nuclear facilities to be built. Anywhere at all. Ever.

On this last point, Greenpeace, Friends of the Earth and the Green Party are all agreed: we DON'T NEED nuclear power. It is not green, it is not cheap and it is not a solution to climate change; it is merely very, very profitable for a wealthy few. We can transition to truly safe, renewable sources of energy without it.

CHAPTER SIX

FIRE II: POISONOUS TECH

The fact that an opinion has been widely held is no evidence whatever that it is not utterly absurd.

Bertrand Russell, *Marriage and Morals*

In this chapter, I'm going to discuss the other end of the spectrum: long-wavelength, low-frequency rays like microwaves and radio waves. The further you go in this direction, the longer the wavelengths and the shorter the frequencies become, till you get to extremely low frequency (ELF) radiation.

Long-wavelength, low-frequency electromagnetic radiation (EMR) has become much more widespread in the past few years and is affecting many of us in powerful ways of which we may be completely unaware.

JEREMY'S STORY

Jeremy was twenty-nine when he first consulted me, a dynamic young entrepreneur running a successful business from home. Having been someone who went to the gym five times a week and worked long hours with no ill effects, he had within a few short months become sick and exhausted. He complained of a constant headache, specifically 'a sensation of unbearable pressure inside the head', dizziness, fatigue and most of all a worrying cognitive decline: 'I can't think straight!' he said, naturally alarmed. 'It's like my brain is full of cotton wool and my thoughts don't make it through. I can't work properly now; I'm in a thick mental fog.'

Jeremy's diet was excellent. Still, I measured all his nutrient levels and also checked he had no chemical toxins in his system. All clear: he was well-nourished, biochemical tests were fine and toxicology tests negative. Physical examination was normal. So, what was going on? I asked Jeremy if anything had changed in his life or his lifestyle in the preceding year. He couldn't think of anything. Then I began asking awkward questions, such as:

Do you have a wi-fi router on your desk? How far from your body is it? Do you hold your mobile phone next to your head? How many hours a day do you spend talking on it? Do you carry it in your pocket when you're out and about? On aeroplane mode or just on? Do you use a laptop computer on your lap or do you put it on the desk?

It turned out that Jeremy's office was in his bedroom, so his devices were pulsing out electromagnetic radiation at him all night long as well as during the day. He was on the mobile phone for his business about six or seven hours a day and he did hold the phone to his head. He also had a wi-fi router on his desk only a foot or two from his body. And he did sit with his laptop on his lap (it is called a laptop, after all, so why wouldn't you?) and he travelled with his phone in his pocket, fully turned on. In relation to this I asked him an even more difficult question; did he have a girlfriend, and how were things going between them? I apologised for asking this, but, I explained, it was important.

Jeremy did have a long-term girlfriend and they had been trying for a baby, unsuccessfully, for nearly two years. She already had a child from a previous relationship, so she knew she was fertile. Had he done a sperm test? Yes, he had, and the result had been very poor. The few sperm he did produce were misshapen and could not swim. He hadn't connected this unfortunate situation with his other symptoms.[1]

Mobile phones, laptops and wi-fi routers give out electromagnetic radiation (EMR), which is at the opposite end of the EM spectrum from nuclear radiation but, as I'll show in this chapter, is equally harmful. Jeremy's phone and wi-fi router were irradiating his head, while his laptop on his lap was irradiating his testes, prostate, bladder and bowel, as was his phone when it was in his pocket. These are massively inconvenient facts and we would all rather it was not so. (Bowel cancer, which used to be thought of as a disease of the elderly, is now increasing rapidly among the young – defined as people under 50 – while actually declining among the over-50s. The studies demonstrating this[2] all speculate about some putative 'lifestyle' factor that may be making the difference, without naming the most likely culprit: the mobile phone in the pocket.)

Jeremy was initially devastated, then sceptical. How do I know you are right, he asked? Well, I could have given him thousands of published papers with the relevant evidence, a few of which I'll quote in this section, but he said he would prefer direct experience. So, he booked himself on an adventure holiday that was out in the wilds, in the woods, far away from all electronic devices. For two weeks. On his return he reported that within two or three days of the trip his brain had begun to clear; he could think straight again. By the end of the first week his energy was back and his headaches and dizziness were gone. During the second week he felt better than he had for a long time; he felt back to normal.

But then he had to return to his flat. Within twenty-four hours he was really ill again, with all the same symptoms. Then he turned off the wi-fi, the laptop and the phone; he unplugged everything. Within forty-eight hours he was better again. But, he complained at our second consultation, not unreasonably, a person couldn't live like that, cut off from all their friends and work contacts. Of course not. Luckily, he didn't have to. I explained to him the methods I'll describe at the end of this chapter, by which one can stay safely protected from EMR in the home while remaining in touch with friends, family and colleagues and still able to access the internet. It can be done, using hard-wired ethernet cables for the laptop instead of wi-fi, getting air tubes to connect to the phone so that it can remain at a distance from your head, using speakerphone setting when talking, putting the phone on aeroplane mode when travelling and perhaps getting a shielding case for it. And disabling Bluetooth and every other app that you aren't using at that moment, on both phone and laptop and all other devices.

There is much more that can be done and some of it, I'll freely admit, is a damn nuisance. But Jeremy felt it was worth it; some years later his business is booming, he remains very well, his sperm have recovered too, and he has become a father. He uses his phone more safely now, but he also uses it less. His work colleagues know that he is not always at the end of the phone; they just have to leave him a message if he's not answering. No-one is indispensable, no matter how high-powered; no-one needs to be available 24/7.

Some people with electro-hyper-sensitivity have more and worse problems than Jeremy; symptoms can include speeding heart rate, vertigo, flushing, temper attacks, anxiety, tinnitus, body aches and most of the symptoms often labelled as fibromyalgia. More and more doctors are accepting the reality of this, although there is a long way to go.[3]

Jeremy is one of the canary people, as in the canaries down the mine that died when the oxygen ran out, therefore giving the miners advance warning that it was not safe to proceed. His symptoms come under the general heading of 'electro-sensitivity' (ES) or 'electro-hypersensitivity' (EHS – the terms tend to be used interchangeably), from which an estimated 4 per cent of the population suffer.[4] He had one of the milder cases, in the sense that, as soon as he was away from the source of the problem, he recovered. Many people, we could call them those with electro-**hyper**sensitivity, do not really recover, and continue to react badly to even very tiny EM inputs such as a simple electric current; their lives become extremely difficult.

ES/EHS are directly comparable to, and often coexist with, multiple chemical sensitivity (MCS). People with MCS have been damaged by excess exposure to toxic chemicals such as those we encountered in chapters 1 to 4, and thereafter react with severe symptoms to any exposure, even to tiny amounts of chemicals, which healthy people cannot even smell. In both cases, the sufferers are canary people and, in both cases, their suffering stands as a warning to all of us that it is not safe to proceed. It's them today, the rest of us tomorrow, if we don't change direction and make our use of this technology a whole lot safer.

What Is EMR and Where Is It Coming From?

Electromagnetic radiation (EMR), also known as electromagnetic fields (EMFs), means forms of radiation that have low frequencies and long wavelengths; in other words, they are at the opposite end of the EM spectrum from nuclear radiation. Common terms you will hear in this context are: radiofrequency radiation (RFR), microwaves (MW), very low frequency (VLF) and extremely low frequency (ELF) radiation. It's non-ionising radiation; unlike nuclear radiation, it does not have the power to directly knock electrons out of atoms and molecular structure. At least, that's the official view. The picture that's emerging, however, is not quite so reassuring.

The EMR spectrum includes radar, microwaves, mobile phone signals (1G – analogue; 2G – Global System for Mobile Communications (GSM); 3G; 4G; 5G and beyond – the 'G' stands for generation) and many variants of wi-fi. Like so many other toxins we've encountered in this book, it began life as a weapon. In the case of EMR, during the Cold War. This EMR is coming out of your microwave oven, your mobile phone, your digital enhanced cordless telecommunications (DECT) phone and its base (but not from your old-fashioned hard-wired landline), your wi-fi router,[5] tablets like the iPad, your laptop computer when connected to wi-fi, your Bluetooth earbuds and headphones,[6] your induction hob[7] and from fluorescent lights. It's coming from fitness trackers, a wireless mouse, gaming consoles, 'smart' meters, 'smart' TVs and all devices enabling the 'Internet of Things'.

Most worryingly, EMR is coming out of DECT and wi-fi electronic baby monitors, which parents use to check on their babies when they're in a different room. It is simpler and safer to keep the baby in the same room with you, even when asleep; babies need human contact and they don't need to be irradiated. In hospitals, EMR is also emitted by the electric engines of incubators for sick/premature newborn babies, which are very near the baby's body. The EMF levels in incubators have been shown to be high enough to suppress the production of the essential hormone melatonin from the pineal gland.[8] Melatonin, as we'll see below, is a vital anti-cancer substance and both the sick babies and their nurses are being exposed to EMR that is suppressing it.

Outside the home, EMR is being emitted from the mobile phone masts (cell phone towers/base stations) that have been springing up around the country like mushrooms after rain and with about as much consultation. These masts are pulsing out high levels of EM radiation and there is evidence that people living close to them are suffering increased risks of cancer, especially breast and brain tumours.[9] They are also – wait for it – more at risk of headaches, skin rashes, sleep disturbances, depression, decreased libido, increased rates of suicide, concentration problems, dizziness, memory changes, tremors and more.[10] Anyone with metal implants in their body is even more at risk from living near such a mast because metal amplifies the EMR signal. And that includes those with metal fillings in their teeth.[11]

Overhead power lines are another source of intense EM radiation, and proximity to them has been associated with significantly increased risk of childhood leukaemia.[12] This could be a double whammy; the effect may be coming both from the high electric and magnetic fields and the fact that these power lines attract and concentrate radioactive particles and other pollutants.[13]

How Does EMR Damage Our Bodies?

One biological mechanism for all these symptoms and sicknesses is thought to be 'oxidative stress'; when the blood of people living near mobile phone masts is analysed, it shows an increase in toxic 'free radicals', a decrease in the healthy antioxidants that we depend on to defend us from those free radicals and increased 'lipid peroxidation' (which means our fat becoming oxidised in precisely the way that leads to heart disease) as well as damage to our genes.[14] EMR actually causes breaks in the strands of our DNA,[15] and this can lead to cell death or to mutations that, as we've seen, result in cancer, birth defects and infertility. Martin Blank, PhD, points out that the DNA molecule, extraordinary structure that it is, is in the form of a coiled coil and thus acts as a 'fractal antenna' – it picks up most wavelengths of EMFs, which may partly explain why EMFs seem to target DNA.[16] And the technology is changing all the time; when 2G changed to 3G, the rate of resultant breaks in DNA increased ten-fold.[17] That was fifteen years ago; by the time equivalent studies on 5G and 6G are published – if they ever see the light of day – what new horrors will they show?

What we do know, and we knew it before the advent of 5G, is that there seems to be one underlying mechanism in our cells that explains the oxidative stress, the DNA strand breaks and all the other biological problems resulting from EMF exposure. It concerns calcium, an important mineral that is not only needed for making bones; it also has a role in 'cell signalling', the way our cells send messages to each other. Normally, there is vastly more calcium in our body fluids than there is inside our cells; calcium is primarily an 'extra-cellular' mineral – it lives outside our cells (in contrast to magnesium, which is mostly 'intra-cellular', meaning it lives inside our cells). However, there is a route for such minerals to enter and exit our cells, through the cell's membrane.

Our cell membranes do not let ions (charged atoms) like calcium into the cell freely; such ions can only get in via very specific channels. These channels are made of protein molecules folded into the shape of pores, occurring at intervals along the cell membrane. Think of the wall around a medieval city, with guarded gates at intervals. The 'guard at the gate' for some of these cell membrane ion channels is electrical; a slight change in electrical charge, which in nature would be occasional, subtle and for a 'purpose' to do with cell signalling, is the password that will allow a few calcium ions in. These channels are called voltage gated ion channels (VGICs) and the calcium ones (VGCCs) can allow calcium both into and out of the cell. In the presence of microwaves, wi-fi and mobile-phone radiation, these channels are forced wide open and calcium then floods into the cell.

Calcium flooding into cells is a very bad thing; remember, calcium should live primarily outside the cell. Numerous scientists have now documented the many and varied biochemical catastrophes that result from all this calcium getting inside cells, where it doesn't belong.[18] Pre-eminent among these scientists is Dr Martin Pall, who says that 'oxidative stress, single and double stranded breaks in DNA, blood–brain barrier breakdown, depressed melatonin levels and sleep disruption, cancer, male and female infertility, immune and neurological and cardiac dysfunction … including sudden cardiac death' can all be fully explained by the action of EMR on those vital channels, the voltage-gated calcium channels.[19] VGICs also exist for potassium and sodium ions. All three play important roles in cell metabolism and neural communications in the brain and central nervous system.[20]

But surely, I hear you ask, they wouldn't let this technology be unleashed on the public if it could harm our health? Surely they must have tested it first? The answers are, respectively, yes they would and no they haven't. Governments are very closely financially tied up with the tech industries whom they are supposed to regulate and from whom they receive large amounts of money – in taxes and possibly in other forms. We'll examine the implications of this later on.

Shortly we'll look further at what EMR does to our bodies and brains in terms of common diseases. First of all, we have to remember that we ourselves are electrical beings. Our nerve messages are transmitted electrically between brain and body, and within the brain. The beating of our heart is controlled electrically. All our cells 'speak' to each other by signals that are both chemical and electrical. So, any changes in the electromagnetic fields surrounding us are bound to affect us. We evolved in the earth's natural electromagnetic field, pretty much unchanged for millions of years, and we can be in contact with that again by standing barefoot on the grass or on a beach. You feel the difference, the sense of physical 'rightness', at once.

However, most of us now live indoors, surrounded by electromagnetic influences that are completely new in human (or animal or plant) history. Dr Martin Blank says the levels are millions of times stronger than natural background radiation.[21] Dr Devra Davis says that 'the current recommended maximum exposure guidance level for human-made radio frequency radiation that is used worldwide is over a trillion times the natural level that we were exposed to less than a hundred years ago.'[22] Professor Olle Johansson of the Karolinska Institute, Stockholm, says that today's maximum limits are too high by a factor of 10^{15} to 10^{18}. Those are hard numbers to get our heads round: 10^{12} is a trillion; 10^{15} is a 'one' followed by 15 noughts. Ten to the power of 18 is just – unimaginably huge.[23] Furthermore, these EM waves, of frequencies that our bodies are not evolved to cope with, are irregular, pulsed, square and spiky as opposed to smooth, regular sine waves like those we get from sunlight.[24]

EMR makes some people, like Jeremy, ill in an obvious and immediate way. But in other people it does damage that is invisible until it manifests in a life-threatening illness like cancer.[25] Unlike Jeremy, the people who get these life-threatening illnesses don't usually feel anything when being exposed to EMR. Or, if they do, they don't associate their symptoms with the exposure; after all, EMR is part of everyday life now. And often there may be quite a time lag (called 'latency') between the cause of the serious illness and its appearing, which makes the connection harder to see. That is why we need better, independently funded, peer-reviewed studies, as the Big Tech/Telecoms industry and governments have been funding studies, by their own scientists, to show no consistent effects. The tobacco industry did exactly the same thing – and got away with it for fifty years.[26]

To Which Diseases Is EMR Contributing?

Just before I launch into the illnesses that EMR can cause, contribute to or exacerbate, let me remind you: there are ways to protect ourselves from EMR, both outdoors and in our own homes. So, there is no need to panic. I'll describe these methods of self-protection at the end of the chapter. But, as I said in relation to nuclear radiation, we can only protect ourselves from a danger if we know it's there. Let's start at the beginning: making – or not making – babies.

Fertility

Fertility is falling rapidly everywhere and the effects of mobile-phone radiation on sperm quality is a major factor in this trend.[27] The human ovum (egg) is obviously harder to study, but we can reasonably assume that similar damage – fragmentation of the DNA[28] – is occurring there too, if a switched-on mobile phone is carried in the pocket or if a laptop is used on the lap, connected to wi-fi. And when women exposed to mobile-phone radiation do manage to conceive, they have a significantly greater risk of miscarriage than women less exposed.[29]

Neurodegeneration

Brain cells (neurones) are directly damaged by EMFs; studies find that just a couple of hours of mobile-phone exposure causes brain damage that looks, under the microscope, exactly like what we see in the brains of people with Alzheimer's disease.[30] It seems that EMR encourages the production of beta-amyloid protein in the brain, a sticky, unnatural, distorted form of protein that is found in the brains of people with Alzheimer's disease.[31] A study in Switzerland found that people who lived very close to electric power lines had a greater mortality from Alzheimer's and the longer they had lived there the higher the risk. People who lived more than 600 metres away were a lot safer.[32]

EMR causes disruption to the blood–brain barrier, an important set of specialised blood vessels that protect the brain from any substances in the body that shouldn't get into the brain. EMR increases the barrier's permeability, so that it leaks (leaky brain, like leaky gut). This means that any toxins in the body will have full access to the brain. This has been known for a long time; it was first described back in the 1970s by Dr Allan Frey, and again more recently both by Frey and other researchers.[33] This damage to the blood–brain barrier is seen even when – as is usually the case – the EMR causes no heating effect in the body's tissues. This fact matters a lot because the telecoms industry's main argument for the alleged safety of EMR is its claim that damage can only result when/if the body gets heated by the radiation. But countless studies show that heating effects are irrelevant; the blood–brain barrier, along with other parts of our anatomy, sustains damage from the non-thermal effects of EMR.[34]

We know that the blood–brain barrier is disrupted in other neurological diseases too, such as Parkinson's disease;[35] could mobile-phone radiation be one of the contributing factors here, too? Another neurodegenerative disease, motor neurone disease (also known as ALS, amyotrophic lateral sclerosis, and as Lou Gehrig's disease) is becoming commoner and occurring in younger and younger people. Epidemiologist Dr Sam Milham noticed that there were three cases of ALS among a team of just fifty-five professional footballers, young athletes at the peak of physical fitness. That's a rate seventy-five times higher than the national average; it's a rare disease, though getting less rare.[36] What Dr Milham discovered was that the physiotherapists who worked with the team used all sorts of electrical and electronic devices to treat the inevitable muscular injuries that occurred during the course of playing. Could there be a connection?

Sadly, all three players have now died, as has a young basketball star, Melissa Jo Erickson, who used assorted electrical devices for the same purpose.[37] If you look her up, you'll see what an amazing basketball player and much-loved person she was, but you won't see anything about the role of EMR in causing the tragic disease that killed her. Despite the vast amount of evidence in the public domain, including all the references quoted in this chapter, this crucial information still hasn't made it from the learned journals into the mainstream media.

Mental Health

Mental health can also be impacted by the damaging effects of EMR on the blood–brain barrier. Depression and other psychiatric problems are linked with exposure to EMR[38], as is impaired cognitive function in children.[39] Time spent on electronic devices seems to increase the rate of both depression and suicide among teenagers.[40] Children are not just smaller overall, they also have thinner skulls and their brains and bone marrow absorb more electromagnetic radiation than those of adults.[41] More on pollution's effects on mental health in Appendix I.

Leukaemia in Children

We have seen that both nuclear fallout and the EM fields generated by high-voltage power lines increase the risk of childhood leukaemia.[42] Exposure to EMR via mobile phones can have the same effect, as can proximity to a mobile phone mast.[43] The BioInitiative Working Group has gathered hundreds of studies confirming this link and other damage done to us by EMR.[44] Among adults, occupational exposure to high EMR levels has also been found to increase the risk of developing leukaemia.[45]

Asthma in Children

It appears that air pollution is not the only factor in childhood asthma. If a mother is exposed to EMFs while her child is in the womb, that child has an increased risk of developing asthma.[46]

Autism in Children

You may remember that in chapter 2 I discussed the role of toxic heavy metals in the genesis of autism. Well, it seems that EMR plays a role too, and its role may be connected with that of metals such as mercury. Metals in the body attract EMR, and possibly amplify it, and, it seems, EMR interferes with the body's ability to rid itself of heavy metals.[47] Babies exposed in the womb to EMR, from their mother's mobile phone or other sources, may be more at risk of autism, which is vastly commoner than it was even a generation ago.[48] We are beginning to understand the mechanisms by which EMR may contribute to autism, and they include oxidative stress as described above, with associated damage to mitochondria (organelles that produce energy in our cells), cell membranes and more.[49]

ADHD in Children

Hyperactivity and other behavioural difficulties in children may, it seems, be linked to both prenatal and postnatal exposure to EMFs.[50] On the positive side, I've found in my own practice some ways to improve the experience and behaviour of children with autism and ADHD, not only with nutrition, diet and detox but also by removing them from an EMF-filled environment. When parents take their children out into the countryside, especially in the woods, as far as possible from EMR, they do calm down.[51] (But beware the occasional mobile phone mast disguised as a tree – I kid you not.)

Childhood Obesity

This is a surprising one. Obesity at any age has many contributory causes, of course, including bad diet, lack of exercise and, as we saw in chapters 1 and 3, pesticides and plastics. But here again it seems that EMR makes a contribution, even before birth. The more EMFs a pregnant woman is exposed to, the greater the chance that the child will suffer from obesity.[52]

Brain Tumours

In 1979 I was on the neurology ward at Chapel Allerton Hospital in Leeds. I had been summoned, along with a great number of other medical students, to see a patient of forty-four with a brain tumour. The poor man in the bed was surrounded. The consultant was excited; this was very unusual. He described the man's symptoms and how they correlated with what had been seen on the brain scan – in the traditional ward-round fashion of the day, which was as if the patient wasn't there. 'Take note,' said the consultant, 'you are all very lucky to be seeing this. It is exceedingly rare, and I expect you won't see another case like it in your training, or even in the rest of your careers.'

Oh, how I wish he had been right. Unfortunately, there has been a substantial rise in the incidence of brain tumours in recent years,[53] and there is a lot of evidence to suggest that exposure to mobile phone radiation is the reason why.[54] I've cited only a few of the hundreds of published papers on this and you can find many more in the 2012 BioInitiative Working Group report, compiled by a hardworking group of concerned scientists, at www.bioinitiative.org. Some of the studies show that the tumours grow on the same side of the head where the person holds their phone. Some show effects from cordless landlines as well as mobiles. Most show worse effects in heavy users of mobile phones and especially in those who have been using them heavily for ten years or more. A Swedish review showed that those who began using a mobile phone before the age of twenty were five times more likely to develop a brain tumour later on than those who hadn't.[55] (Sweden adopted mobile phone use before most other countries, so they were able to make the comparison sooner.)

These days, every teenager is using a mobile phone, and using it regularly; that's a scary thought for their parents. Depending where the EMR comes out of the phone, it may target the brain, the throat or the parotid salivary gland in the cheek; studies have found an increase in parotid gland tumours on the side of the face where users hold their mobile phone.[56] They have also found, associated with long-term (over ten years') use of mobile and cordless phones, an increase in acoustic neuroma, a tumour of the eighth cranial nerve that takes messages between the ear and the brain, enabling us to hear and to keep our balance.[57] That's in addition to the increase in occurrence of glioma, a tumour of the 'supporting cells' in the brain.[58]

Breast Cancer

As you'll know if you've read this far in the book, there are many factors contributing to the explosive rise of breast cancer in the past few decades. Now we have to add radiation from mobile phones and masts to the impact of pesticides, plasticiser chemicals, synthetic hormones and heavy metals.[59] Women who work in electrical industries are especially likely to get breast cancer,[60] but men are not immune to it either; a cluster of men with breast cancer have been found among male electrical workers.[61]

How does this happen? The most likely mechanism is that, as we've seen in the context of babies in incubators, EMR suppresses production of the hormone melatonin by the pineal gland in the brain. Melatonin is vital not just for helping us get to sleep at night, but also for protecting the reproductive system; it prevents puberty from happening too early and it prevents all sorts of cancers from occurring in the reproductive organs, which include the breasts. Not only does the blue light coming from mobile phone screens suppress melatonin, so does the EMR. Double whammy – again. Melatonin is a powerful antioxidant, which turns out to prevent (and slow down the growth of) all tumours, not just reproductive ones; suppressing its production by our addiction to mobile phones seems like a very bad idea. No doubt yet other mechanisms will also be discovered by which EMR causes (or speeds up the progression of) cancer, but the experimental and epidemiological evidence is very clear that it does so.[62]

Nosebleeds, cataracts, tinnitus, insomnia, abnormal heart rhythms, accelerated ageing and raised blood pressure[63] are also on the list of ailments to which EMR can contribute,[64] as of course is electro-sensitivity, as described above. But I won't go on. I'll tell you instead about a young boy whom I was able to help considerably by reducing his exposure to EMR.

STEPHAN'S STORY

Stephan was twelve when his mother brought him to see me in 2018, with a diagnosis of epilepsy. His parents and teachers were concerned about the medication he'd been prescribed because it was making him fall asleep in class; but on the other hand, the fits did need to be suppressed because they were dangerous. We don't usually know the root cause of epilepsy, but we can sometimes identify triggers that set off a seizure. Often, I've found the trigger is hypoglycaemia, due to missing meals (and/or eating excess sugar, which allows the blood glucose level to rise abruptly and then, as a result of insulin action, fall too low or too fast). However, Stephan was eating fine; the trigger turned out to be a combination of three main sources of electromagnetic radiation. There was wi-fi at school, there were the electronic screens on which he played games all the time at home and there was his mobile phone. It was very noticeable, said Stephan's mother, that the fits were worse and more frequent towards the end of the school week, and particularly bad when he had been indoors for a long time at home, playing on his screens.

Stephan wanted to get off his drugs (they weren't working anyway, despite making him sleepy) so he agreed, reluctantly, to go 'cold turkey' from his electronic devices. For two whole weeks he had no screen time at all and didn't use his phone; unfortunately, though, we couldn't turn off the wi-fi at school, which is doing untold harm to children's mental and physical health.[65] During that fortnight Stephan had only one fit, at the end of a school week. Then it was the Easter holidays and Stephan spent the days outside, cycling and playing football with his mates. He had no fits at all and since then has been able to wean himself slowly off the drugs, so he is more awake and able to focus at school.

He has dropped the screen games, having discovered that he prefers real games outdoors with real companions; he has joined two local sports teams. He is using his mobile phone only on speakerphone, has a shielding case around it and limits his use. Mostly he sends texts, and he sometimes uses shielding gloves to protect his hands from the radiation. (I'll give you a list at the end of the chapter of companies that sell these shielding products.) By the age of fifteen, Stephan no longer considered himself epileptic, although technically he is, and still has the occasional (milder) fit after a week of wi-fi exposure at school. He never gets them during the holidays and he has asked to be excused from computer science at school.

I have seen other epileptic children in whom fits were triggered by proximity to a mobile phone mast. Dr Gerard Hyland of Warwick University noticed the same phenomenon; a child in whom fits increased from two per month to eight per day when close to a mast.[66] I have had to advise families to move house in this situation, which is a big ask, and it's getting harder and harder to find anywhere that's not too near a mast. However, the conventional medical approach, even now, is to dismiss such claims as 'psychosomatic'. In response, Dr Hyland points out that in the vicinity of such masts there is also reduced growth in pine trees and damage to DNA (chromosomes/genes) in plants and in cows. As Jonathan Mantle asks: 'Could pine trees pretend? Did plants dissimulate? Might cows be imagining things?'[67]

Stephan is relatively lucky. Wi-fi at school was fatal for the teenager Jenny Fry. For about three years she had been suffering from severe fatigue, headaches and bladder problems whenever she was near wi-fi routers. Her parents removed wi-fi from their house and then she was fine at home. Unfortunately, though, her school had wi-fi in most classrooms, and refused to let Jenny go elsewhere to work; in fact, when she asked, they put her in detention – in a room with wi-fi. Jenny became more and more ill, more and more desperate, and in June 2015 she took her own life, leaving notes explicitly stating that it was because of the wi-fi; she couldn't take it any longer.[68] Her mother, Debra Fry, continues to campaign for the removal of wi-fi from schools and nurseries; she is a brave and determined person whom I am privileged to have met on at least two occasions. Like Ella Kissi-Debrah's mother, Rosamund, whom we encountered in chapter 4, she is turning personal grief into care for others, trying to prevent further tragedies.

Is This a Real Problem?

Electro-sensitivity has been known for some decades, but it is becoming both more common and more severe as the density of the 'electro-smog' surrounding us increases. Perhaps the most famous person to suffer from it is Gro Brundtland,[69] three times prime minister of Norway, who is a qualified doctor and has a master's degree in public health from Harvard. In 1998, she became director of the World Health Organization. In 2002, having banned mobile phones from her office in Geneva because they made her feel so ill, she was criticised for 'scaring the public' and, she said, for 'telling the truth about my illness'.[70] A few months later, sooner than expected, she left her post at the WHO.

As with many new illnesses, patients are not always believed; their symptoms are dismissed as a 'nocebo' effect, meaning that they are imagining the symptoms and/or that EMR is causing them. ('Nocebo' means an imagined harm, from the Latin 'I shall harm', just as 'placebo' means an imagined benefit, from the Latin 'I shall please'.) But there have been plenty of controlled studies showing that, for the people who suffer from it, electro-sensitivity is all too real,[71] and more and more medical scientists internationally are acknowledging this.[72] Furthermore, I was taught in medical school: 'Listen to the patient: they are telling you the diagnosis.' Even, I would add, if the diagnosis is not yet in the medical textbooks.

If a person feels ill in the vicinity of EMR, it is likely to be the EMR that is causing the sensation, not a 'nocebo' effect. There is a growing list of conditions that start off being dismissed as imaginary and will end up being finally, reluctantly, acknowledged as real by the medical profession. Chronic fatigue syndrome/ME, multiple chemical sensitivity, aerotoxic syndrome as well as electro-sensitivity, are some recent examples. One of the arguments always used to dismiss such people as malingerers is that not everyone is made ill by exposure to synthetic chemicals or EMR. Well, of course. We're all biologically different, with differing vulnerabilities/ predispositions; everyone knows somebody's grandma who smoked sixty a day and lived to one hundred. That doesn't mean smoking doesn't cause lung cancer. But the tobacco industry certainly used that argument – that not all smokers die of lung cancer – to claim that their products were totally safe.

The tech industry is doing the same thing today. They are also funding dodgy studies (studies that are methodologically flawed) to try to show 'no effect' or a 'nocebo' effect. There is a very painful description in Mantle and Stein's book *The Microwave Delusion* of Brian Stein's experience, as an electro-sensitive person, of innocently choosing to participate in one such trial in order, he assumed, to help advance the research and thus help other sufferers. The study was commissioned by the UK Health Protection Agency (as then was) – but it turned out to be funded by the mobile phone industry. The EMF exposure to which Brian was subjected during the trial made him very ill, but the trial was rigged in such a way that his experience was not even included in the results.[73]

Many doctors and scientists, however, are now recognising the reality and seriousness, not only of electro-sensitivity but also of all the other risks that electromagnetic radiation poses to us and to all life on earth. In 2020 a group of such expert practitioners signed a concise but thoroughly referenced consensus statement that summarises the science, warns of the dangers and makes sensible recommendations that should be urgently heeded.[74]

Save the Birds, Bees and Trees – Save the Humans Too!

In the context of a book linking environmental issues with human-health issues, it's important to remember that we share most of our DNA with other animal species and indeed with plants. So whatever damages us is likely to damage them, and vice versa. When people talk about 'the environment' they sometimes forget that the environment is not some inanimate place where we live, it is the sum total of all life on earth as well as the mountains and valleys, plains and cities, rivers and oceans that this life occupies. Wildlife conservationists need to be thinking about the impact of EMR on animals and plants – and it is considerable. In a world full of artificial electromagnetic radiation, it is not only we humans who are getting sick and dying.

Colony collapse disorder (CCD) is the term used for the fact that bees – essential pollinators without whom we would have very little to eat – are dying. Whole hives are dying, whole collections of hives.[75] The number of bees is plummeting and so is the number of species of bees. Undoubtedly the overuse of insecticides/pesticides plays an important part, as do habitat loss and climate change, and entomologists are also blaming parasites/mites/viruses. But these parasites/mites/viruses have been around forever; we have to ask, what has so weakened the immune system of the bees that they can no longer fight off these bugs? Maybe when the insecticides don't actually kill the insects, they weaken them so they become more vulnerable to such infections? (A bit like humans.) But it looks as if electromagnetic radiation also has a major role here.

Bees have to be able to forage for nectar and then find their way back to their hive. They do this largely by using the natural electromagnetic field of the earth as their compass. When exposed to the artificial EM field generated by a typical cordless phone, many of them become unable to find their way home.[76] When exposed to mobile-phone radiation, queen bees lay far fewer eggs, the bees' behaviour changes, colony strength declines and, as one researcher says, 'There was neither honey nor pollen in the colony at the end of the experiment'.[77] EM radiation at the level of an ordinary mobile phone alters the development of baby bees[78] and causes the worker bees to emit their alarm call, 'piping' – it's as if they know something is wrong.[79] The decline in the honeybee population is pretty desperate all over the world, and more and more evidence is accruing that the huge rise in EMR is the major cause.[80]

It is not only bees; other insects are being impacted as well. It seems that even very low levels of EMR can inhibit their ability to reproduce[81] as well as to navigate. Most of the scientists who are studying these effects point out that 5G is being rolled out without any prior investigation of its potential damaging effects on ecosystems.[82] By 'ecosystems' they may mean the birds and the bees – but ecosystems of course include humans.

It's important to understand that the EMR that's affecting the bees, birds and humans is everywhere, now, all the time; even when people are not making a call, their phone (unless it's off or in aeroplane mode) is connecting with the nearest mast, so EM signals are flying around all the time – around us and through us. Through our bodies and through those of every other living creature. Birds and bees are trying to find their way through this 'electro-smog' and are dying at alarming rates.[83] EMR from mobile masts is interfering with the reproduction of bird species from white storks[84] to chickens.[85] And this is apart from birds flying into power lines and mobile phone towers and suffering electrocution, which, even as long ago as 2005, was estimated to kill many tens of millions of birds every year.[86] In our gardens, house sparrows are declining drastically due to EMR;[87] the higher the intensity of EMR from neighbouring base stations (mobile phone towers), the fewer sparrows were found,[88] and the correlation was 'highly significant', meaning it couldn't have been a result of chance.

Tadpoles doing their level best to become frogs are seriously affected; in one experiment, among tadpoles located 140 metres from a mobile phone mast, 90 per cent died. Among the tadpoles in the same place but protected from the EM radiation by a Faraday bag, only 4.2 per cent died; the rest successfully turned into frogs[89] (but not princes). Yes, you can get a Faraday bag to carry your phone in when you're not using it; info at end of chapter – it's the same thing that's used to prevent theft of the RFID signal of car key fobs, and to stop your credit card being scanned by criminals in a crowd as you're walking along a busy high street. It used to be thought that only animals with poor vision used the earth's magnetic field for navigating, but it turns out that the orientation even of animals who can see quite well, such as the humble wood mouse, is altered by EM fields.[90] How about us? Could human orientation abilities be impacted by EMR? We don't know – but indirectly they certainly are, in that we have outsourced our sense of direction to GPS/SatNav.

You may have noticed that whales and other marine mammals are increasingly getting 'beached'; stranded where they are not meant to be. Unless they can be found in time and pushed back into the water, they die. Could EMR be the explanation? It looks possible. It is already known that solar storms, which disrupt the earth's electromagnetic field, can lead to such strandings.[91] We know that whales use a 'magnetic sense' to navigate over thousands of miles, as do migrating birds, and that artificially generated EM fields, such as those created by 'EM surveys' to look for petrol under the ocean, risk sending them way off course.[92] In a study just released, scientists express concern that 'anthropogenic' (created by us) radiofrequency radiation is leading to more strandings of cetaceans – that's dolphins, whales and porpoises.[93] Other scientists are worrying about the effect of undersea electric cables on the movement of fish and other sea animals.[94]

Trees and other plants can be severely impacted by EMR. Studies have shown that trees near mobile phone masts are damaged and eventually die, and that the side of the tree facing the mast is significantly more damaged than the side facing away.[95] How are the trees in your local park doing? Maybe have a look. If one looks poorly, you might want to check where the nearest mast is in relation to it. Plants experience EMR as a stressor: they have a 'stress response' when exposed to it. Studies on tomato plants show that this is mediated in much the same way as in humans; calcium flooding into the plant's cells, as described above.[96] And the result is that the plants produce lots of free radicals and don't grow very well.[97] EMR causes them to suffer from 'oxidative stress' just like we do.[98] Tests on edible plants such as wheat, amaranth and mung beans have shown that seedlings don't germinate properly when surrounded by EMR.[99] And in a five-year-long study, agricultural wheat production was found to be lowered when the wheat was grown underneath high voltage power lines.[100]

If all this touches you and/or you are a wildlife conservationist/activist or have a friend who is, the best website for further info is www.wildlifeandwireless.org, created by the Environmental Health Trust in the US. It's full of good info about the science and about actions being taken to make a difference. Think global, act local.

The Fifth Generation – 5G

The fifth generation of wireless technology, 5G, is in some ways different from previous incarnations of EMR technology. It will use 'higher RF frequencies and different modulation, with higher amplitude, rapid data bursts which are expected to cause even greater cellular damage'.[101] But it will not be replacing the existing 4G EMR; it will simply be adding to it. It will include millimetre waves, MMWs, which have been claimed to be safe because they don't penetrate our bodies very far. But the skin, eye and testes are all surface structures, which may indeed be affected, and increases in skin cancers, cataracts and testicular cancer are worrying possibilities.[102] And the sweat glands in our skin may act as antennae, intensifying our exposure.[103] How many studies have been done to make sure it's safe before it's rolled out? Er – none. But many scientists are seriously worried about the potential health risks, including physical pain.[104]

The 'not penetrating very far' element of MMWs is important; these waves can't get through trees, so trees may be felled to allow them through. They can't get through buildings either. Therefore, the telecoms companies are going to create 'base stations with massive MIMO (Multiple Input/Multiple Output) transmitters, and receivers in millions of small cell towers ... installed on structures such as utility poles'.[105] To get them through the walls of your house, these waves will have to be 'beamformed',[106] many frequencies concentrated into a single beam; it will be hard to get away from them, indoors or outdoors.

Why are the telecoms companies doing all this? Simple. They can achieve greater bandwidth and faster connectivity, and enable the 'Internet of Things', without having to invest in laying fibre-optic cables.[107] That's about it; it will be much cheaper for them than physical cables. It's for their profit, not your convenience, and certainly not your health. In fact, our health may be the price we pay for the privilege of being able to turn on our central heating from the other side of town, set the washing machine going remotely or pay with our wristwatch in a shop. Is it really worth it?

There is resistance. At date of writing this (12 Jan 2024), some 304,670 scientists, doctors and ordinary citizens who don't want to be zapped have signed the International Appeal to Stop 5G on Earth and in Space, and the numbers will be higher by the time you read this. You might choose to add your name.[108] After all, there has been no consultation and certainly no informed consent. This is a massive, uncontrolled and unethical experiment on all of us: humans, animals, trees and plants. It goes against the Nuremberg Code. If we don't stop it, 6G and 7G will be upon us before we know it.

Some countries have taken measures to limit EMR exposure;[109] for example, France has banned wi-fi in nurseries and massively reduced its use in schools. Wired internet connections work just fine. But Britain and the US appear to be pressing on regardless. Nevertheless, some UK local councils are fighting for the right to refuse 5G infrastructure in their area. Mendip District Council in Somerset, South West England, is one that has said 'No'.

John William Frank, an experienced epidemiologist and Professor Emeritus at Edinburgh University, is one of many scientists to put in a plea for the Precautionary Principle – a fundamental principle in medicine – to be applied in the case of 5G. (The UK's 'Stewart Report' had already called for the precautionary principle to be applied to mobile-phone use, especially for children, way back in 2000.) Professor Frank and others are calling for a moratorium on this dangerous technology.[110] He has also pointed out[111] that when the industry says, 'there is no conclusive evidence of harm', that is code for saying, 'we haven't done any serious studies and we're not going to'. In medical science, we have an important aphorism: 'Absence of evidence is not evidence of absence.' The onus should be on industry to prove something is safe, rather than on scientists to prove it is lethal.

But it is difficult and risky to challenge any product or activity that makes billions of dollars for the powerful; those doing the challenging may be vilified, mocked, ignored or murdered. People opposing 5G are often mocked and vilified, as Rachel Carson was for campaigning against toxic pesticides in the 1960s. In South America, every year, about 200 environmental activists, trying to preserve the rainforests and other crucial ecosystems, are murdered;[112] they threaten the profits of mining/logging/Big Ag companies. The victims of asbestos, trying to get justice, are still largely being ignored; some are dying today, without compensation. And the scientists who were telling the world that tobacco was dangerous for all those decades received similar treatment;

the industry formed the Tobacco Institute to attack them and fight its corner, using astonishingly corrupt and sophisticated tactics,[113] tactics that the telecoms industry is now emulating.[114] (Their equivalent of the Tobacco Institute in the US is the CTIA, Cellular Telecommunications Industry Association.) They will stop at nothing to protect their profits; it's down to us to protect our health. Governments won't do it, and nor will doctors.

Setting the Standards – Who's Keeping Us Safe?

There are official safety standards for EMR exposure – but how were they created, when and by whom?

The international body that sets the maximum 'safe limits' is ICNIRP, the International Commission on Non-Ionizing Radiation Protection. Its guidelines, originally set in the 1990s, were based on brief experiments, done in the 1980s, on eight rats and five monkeys.[115] These experiments used EMR exposures of only 40–60 minutes' duration and as a 'one-off', even though many people now use their phone throughout the day and for many years. The resultant ICNIRP guidelines ignore the 20,000 plus research papers published since the 1990s that show serious biological effects of EMR.[116] Extraordinarily, the guidelines, although updated in 2020,[117] still don't look at biological effects; ICNIRP only consider 'thermal effects': heating.

Their assumption is that only by heating our body tissues can EMR do us any damage. This is one of fourteen assumptions recently shown to be false, in the way ICNIRP has set its standards.[118] We have seen the damage that EMR can do and most of these effects are 'non-thermal'; they're quite irrespective of temperature rises.[119] ICNIRP seem to be worrying only about burns or electrocution, which are very rare because the EMR we are discussing gives out far less heat energy than nuclear radiation.

Do you remember, in discussing the dangers of nuclear radiation, Professor Chris Busby's analogy of the burning coal? The amount of heat in that hot coal may be the same as that given out by a warm fire, but if it's all concentrated into one spot it does far more damage if you touch it, than if it's spread out evenly through the whole body by just sitting near the fire. Interestingly, the same sort of 'averaging error' has crept into ICNIRP'S calculations. They talk about the Specific Absorption Rate (SAR) of a mobile phone, meaning how much EMR we absorb from it. But they assume that the EMR is spread out evenly over the whole brain. In fact, it isn't. Different parts of the brain have different densities and absorb EMR differently.

Furthermore, how much EMR you absorb from your phone depends on a host of other factors, such as the angle at which you hold it, how far from your head you hold it, how thick your skull is (yes, really) and how far you are from a mast (ironically, the further away you are, the harder the phone has to work to get signal, so you can get more heavily irradiated by your phone in the country than in the town). It has been known for decades that EMR doesn't 'uniformly move through or heat anything' – the early versions of microwave ovens burnt some parts of the food and left other bits raw. That's why they now rotate, to avoid hot spots and cold spots. But, as Dr Devra Davis points out, we can't rotate our brains while we're on the phone.[120] So, we do in fact get hot spots in the brain or other parts of the head/face/throat, where concentrated EMR does the kind of damage I've documented.

There is a SAR rating somewhere on your phone or on the paperwork that came in the box with it, but it is effectively meaningless. (There is also, probably buried deep in the small print, a warning not to hold it too close to your body. But does anybody read that?)

So much for SAR; now, who is SAM? SAM stands for standard anthropomorphic mannequin, the model used to measure EMR absorption and create the SAR rating of your mobile phone. SAM is supposed to represent the standard human body/brain, but, unfortunately, he is far from resembling the average living person. He is 6 foot 2 inches, weighs about 14.3 stone (200 pounds or 91 kilogrammes), and his 'brain' is a bag full of liquid of uniform density; nothing like the human brain. SAM has no muscle or bone, no meninges (the membranes around the brain, where tumours called meningiomas occasionally occur), no cells and no DNA. Crucially, SAM bears no resemblance to a human child.

None of the ICNIRP guidelines take into account that fact that children are quite biologically different from adults and are far more vulnerable to the effects of EMR. It's not just that children are smaller and their skulls are thinner; their brains are growing fast, and between the ages of five and eight they absorb more than twice as much EMR as do adult brains.[121] Some parts of their brains, including their eyes, absorb three times more and their bone marrow absorbs ten times more.[122] This last is especially worrying given the rise in childhood leukaemia,[123] a cancer that originates within the cells of the bone marrow.

The ICNIRP guidelines don't protect any of us, least of all children.[124] Concerns about this have now even reached the esteemed pages of *The Lancet*.[125] The levels of EMR that ICNIRP permits are thousands of times higher than those which have been shown to damage our health.[126] Governments, councils and other authorities often dismiss people's worries about local masts, for instance, by saying 'We've measured, and the levels are within the ICNIRP guidelines'. They may well be within those guidelines and still be very dangerous. Many scientists are now calling for children to be properly protected; for their exposure to EMR to be made 'as low as reasonably achievable' – ALARA.[127] And safer, more realistic guidelines than ICNIRP's can now be found at www.ignir.org; IGNIR stands for International Guidelines on Non-Ionising Radiation and they are based on the peer-reviewed EUROPAEM EMF Guidelines from 2016.[128]

Each country is free to set more stringent standards, if it chooses, to protect its population, and Italy is one that has done so. As a result, Innocenzo Marcolini, a company director who spent five or six hours a day on his mobile phone for twelve years and developed a neurinoma, a tumour on his trigeminal nerve (the fifth cranial nerve), was able to win a court case for compensation. The court agreed that his tumour was most likely caused by his EMR exposure,[129] because it used in evidence the work of independent experts[130] rather than the ICNIRP guidelines. Marcolini had held his phone in his left hand, on the left side of his head, while taking notes with his right hand.[131] His tumour was on the left.

How is it possible that a supposedly independent regulatory organisation like ICNIRP can, in the face of all the evidence, continue to promulgate such useless and dangerous pseudo-safety guidelines? Well, inescapably, it's politics. There is a thing called 'regulatory capture'; it means that the people who are supposed to be impartially regulating, constraining and controlling an industry turn out to be, in fact, part of that industry. There's a 'revolving door' between the industry and the regulatory body; the same people occupy both positions, sometimes alternately, sometimes even at the same time. It's a conflict of interest.

It is not in the interests of the telecoms industry to take on board the overwhelming evidence of the harm their products are doing. It's not that they couldn't improve the tech to make it much safer. They could, but it would cost them a lot of money. And it would constitute an admission that they had got it terribly wrong and open the door to prosecutions. Insurers like Lloyds won't, apparently, insure telecoms companies against possible claims for illness or death caused by mobile phones and the associated technology. And insurers tend to know what's what.

So, based on the views of regulatory agencies like ICNIRP, our governments and local authorities end up 'rubber stamping' most proposed new masts. The industry, ignoring health concerns, ignoring the science that doesn't suit them, continues to claim that decades of substantial research are just 'preliminary findings', that the health concerns are 'not established', not 'proven beyond all reasonable doubt'. The Precautionary Principle gets drowned out by the demand for absolute, conclusive proof of harm, whereas new technologies should first have to prove that they are safe. A person may be innocent till proven guilty, but a new technology isn't.

We didn't wait for 'conclusive proof' before banning CFC aerosols; it looked as if they were destroying the ozone layer above Antarctica, so we stopped their use and now the hole in the ozone layer is closing up. Dr Ignaz Semmelweis, trying to save the lives of mothers and babies in Viennese maternity wards in the nineteenth century, didn't wait for 'absolute proof' that the germs on doctors' hands were causing puerperal fever; he just made the doctors wash their hands and the death rate of mothers and babies plummeted. We didn't even have 'absolute proof' about tobacco and lung cancer, but we eventually – despite that industry's best efforts – took the concerns seriously. And now we do know, absolutely. How many millions of lives could have been saved if we had acted sooner?

Making the Tech Safer: What We Can Do

- We can minimise our use of mobile phones, and particularly restrict children's use. I know it's hard, it's very hard; this tech has been designed to be addictive, like cigarettes. And the desire to stay connected is completely natural. But we have to find other, safer ways to connect. We have to break this love affair with our phones, which is even greater, perhaps, than the love affair with the car that I described in chapter 4.

- Make sure that your phone is on aeroplane mode whenever you're not using it; otherwise, it is continually in touch with the nearest masts and irradiating you just as if you were making a call. When you are speaking on your phone, always use the speakerphone setting. Never hold it to your ear.
- We can get ethernet cables to replace wi-fi with hard-wired internet connections; it works just as well, and often even better. If you have a child at school, you can start a campaign to get the school (if they've installed wi-fi) to replace it with hard-wired internet; they will find that the kids' health, happiness, concentration and academic performance improve. If they haven't got wi-fi but are considering it – prevention is better than cure! To get the connections around the house, you can use dLAN plug-in units, which send the ethernet signal around the house wiring at very low field levels. Then you can get an ethernet connection in every room that has a dLAN box plugged in. Educate the teachers. (Campaign information at the end of the book in Resources.)
- If you use a laptop computer, get a special protective tray or pad to put underneath it (details below), but better still, plug an ethernet cable into its port and disable wi-fi (and Bluetooth). Or just use an old-fashioned PC that stays in one place on your desk. Don't ever put a laptop on your lap or anywhere directly on your body. The same applies to tablets, iPads and similar devices. You can disable all unnecessary apps on your phone, too.
- If you are moving house, do check that you're not going to be living right under a mobile phone mast.
- Before you buy any protective, EMF-shielding clothing, which you might or might not need, buy a meter to measure the EMF levels in your house or flat. The simplest and cheapest is the Acousticom 2, and you can also get a good range of 'Safe and Sound' meters from Safe Living Technologies (see below).
- If you've reduced your exposure as above, but the meter shows high EMFs in your home, it is probably your neighbour's wi-fi and/or mobile phone and/or smart meter. You can get EMF-blocking paint from most of the suppliers listed below; it works, which you can confirm by measuring with your meter before and after. One or two coats will suffice. But it's usually black, so you'll probably then want to paint over it in another colour.

- If you are electro-sensitive, you can buy protective hats, T-shirts and other clothing that reduces your exposure. This is a bit of a 'suck it and see' situation; most of my electro-sensitive patients have found that these clothes make a big difference to how they feel (companies' details below), but there was one electro-hypersensitive lady for whom it didn't help; we're all different.
- When you're out and about, you can put your phone on aeroplane mode, and/or keep it in a Faraday bag, which you can get from one of the suppliers listed below. If you feel that you simply must be contactable at all times – well, challenge that feeling! None of us is indispensable 24/7. Most calls can wait, most people can wait, most of the time.
- You can get an EMR-protective case for your phone, but opinions vary on how much they help; it may depend on the angle at which you hold your phone and from which part of the phone (the antenna) the EMR is being emitted. One advantage that electro-sensitive people have is that they can tell, simply by how they feel, whether the protective equipment is working or not. The rest of us can't, but we should take all possible precautions to protect ourselves anyway, for all the reasons outlined in this chapter.
- Texting is safer than calling because the phone is further away from your head. If you are electro-sensitive, you can get EMR-protective gloves to reduce the unpleasant buzz that ES people feel in their hands when holding a phone.
- Get non-metal air-tube earphones, again to keep the phone at a safe distance from your body. Increasing the phone's distance from your head and/or body even a little way makes a big difference to the amount of EMR you absorb.
- Get rid of your microwave oven. If you want to reheat something from the freezer – anticipate. Take it out the night before. Leave yourself a note. It can be done.
- Some of the companies who make the EMR-protective gear have expert 'EMF surveyors' who will, for a fee, come to your house and measure everything there is to be measured about EMR. They will locate any problem areas in your house and suggest solutions. If they are doing the job properly, they should spend at least a couple of hours with you.

Companies Providing EMR-Protective Products

The charity Electro-Sensitivity UK (www.es-uk.info) has an extensive list of recommended shielding suppliers and EMF surveyors, as well as much other useful info, including a free guide, 'Tips for Reducing EMF Exposure', which you can get from their website. Or, if you're very electro-sensitive and can't look at a computer screen, they will post you a printed copy. So, rather than reproduce their list here, I'll just mention (in alphabetical order) the three companies with which I'm most familiar:

- Beneficial Environments: www.beneficialenvironments.co.uk
- Conscious Spaces: www.consciousspaces.com
- Safe Living Technologies: www.safelivingtechnologies.com/products

These three companies, and probably many others, are run by people who have electro-sensitivity themselves and have been through quite a journey discovering what was wrong and how to fix it. (More information in the Resources section.) Here, briefly, is the story of Tara Williams (her real name, used with her permission); what happened to her and how she came to found her company, Conscious Spaces. In her own words:

> I was very unwell from the age of 19 years. Most of the following decade was spent 90% bedridden and searching for answers. I was eventually diagnosed with ME, Post-Viral Chronic Fatigue Syndrome, Endometriosis and more. Being in constant pain and with significant symptoms, I was told I was probably going to be bedridden for the rest of my life and would never have children.
>
> Within my journey to recovery after learning, studying and researching I found that addressing the 'health' of my environment was key, and a large piece of this puzzle was human-made electromagnetic fields/frequencies in my home and beyond.
>
> Initially, I noticed my body's reactions around radiofrequency: wi-fi routers and mobile phones. My symptoms were anything from my heart racing for hours, to dizziness, brain fog, skin irritation and more.

I thought it was me being more sensitive than the average person due to my health issues.

However, after looking at the science papers, databases and books, discovering that the WHO had classified radiofrequency as a class 2 carcinogen in 2011 and that Sweden had recognised EHS as a functional impairment since the early 2000s, I came to realise that this was in fact a very real problem.

An 'aha' moment came in 2003 when I took a trip to Hippocrates Health Institute in Florida with my husband Darren. Part of the process for the health programme was blood draw on the first and last week as well as Darkfield/Live blood analysis. Darren did the three-week health programme alongside me. In the final week, we were looking at his blood sample on the monitor – there was visual clumping, sticky rouleaux (like coins stuck together in rolls); he had not veered from the programme and he was healthy and had no issues. What was going on?

It came to light that just before this blood was taken, he was on a mobile phone on a business call to the UK for 30 minutes. Wow! This is what non-ionising radiation does to a normal healthy person's cells!

I trained in various healing modalities including Nutritional Therapy (at the Institute for Optimum Nutrition) and EMF surveying with Geovital, based in Austria. This missing piece of the puzzle led me to address EMF 'hygiene', shielding and mitigation as well as rebalancing my body with natural, native EMFs through grounding and other techniques. I regained my health and my life, and this eventually culminated in having my beloved son and, in 2019, starting Conscious Spaces.

Now in my 46th year, this journey of being the 'canary in the coalmine' with EHS has enabled me to help others and also to recognise that these issues, even if you are not currently 'feeling' the effects, are affecting everyone; indeed, all biological life right down to cellular level – we are all electromagnetic beings!

Tara Williams, 2023.

CHAPTER SEVEN

INDOOR POLLUTION: A TOUR OF YOUR HOUSE

Home is where one starts from.

T.S. Eliot, 'East Coker'

Pollution – there's a lot of it about, as you'll know if you've read this far. With air pollution especially, we tend to think of it as being outdoors; mostly traffic fumes. Our home, we expect, should be a sanctuary away from all that, a safe place. And it can be. But indoor pollution is a reality too, and it is putting our health and our children's health at risk. Here's the good news, however: once we know what the sources of indoor pollution are – when we've identified the surprising poisonings of everyday life – we can get rid of them. Simply and permanently. And since we spend 90 per cent of our time indoors, dealing with indoor pollution can make a huge difference to our health, and quickly, too.

The purpose of this chapter is to alert you to the toxic substances that are lurking in your kitchen cupboards, your bathroom cabinets, your living room and your bedroom, and to suggest safe alternatives to these substances. We know now why this matters; we're seeing sky-rocketing rates of chronic, degenerative illnesses that were rare or unknown a century or two ago,[1] and much of this is due to the synthetic chemicals we've manufactured and that our bodies are not equipped to deal with. All the problematic substances I'm going to discuss in this chapter are synthetic, artificial, alien to our biochemistry. Most of them are petrochemicals and many have been labelled as carcinogenic (cancer-inducing), teratogenic (they damage babies in the womb) or endocrine-disrupting (they mess with your hormones). Or all three. Yet you can buy them in any supermarket or chemist.

Furthermore, most of these chemicals are lipophilic – they dissolve in fat. So, once inside our bodies, they are stored in fatty tissue (meaning women are more at risk because they have a higher fat-to-muscle ratio than men) and they make a beeline for the organ that has the highest concentration of fat: the brain. This means they are implicated in mental as well as physical disease. They can penetrate the skin as well as the lungs, and they can go through our cell membranes (because these too are made of fat) and get access to every organ, every cell of the body. Children are more at risk because they are smaller and have a faster breathing rate and thinner skin. But the person most at risk from these handy, familiar, innocent-looking but toxic everyday products is, again, the unborn baby.[2]

So, let's have a look at what these chemicals are and learn how we can avoid unintentionally poisoning ourselves and our kids. Let's start with the kitchen. What's under the sink?

In the Kitchen

Cleaning Chemicals

These include detergents, disinfectants, washing-up liquid, laundry powders, surface cleaners, all-purpose cleaners (sprays are worse than cream cleaners because you inhale more of them), stain removers, window cleaners, furniture polish, oven cleaners, anti-bacterial sprays, anti-bacterial wipes and more. Please, read some of the ingredients lists – find a magnifying glass if necessary! If you haven't got at least A-level chemistry, it looks like gobbledygook, but it's chemical names. You can look them up; there is a publicly available 'data sheet' online for every chemical made, although it tends to describe just the acute effects of accidentally inhaling or swallowing a large amount, rather than the long-term effects of daily, low-dose exposure, which is what I'm worrying about. But it gives you an idea.

Here is just part of a typical ingredients list from a common brand of stain remover for carpets and upholstery: subtilisin (an enzyme, used also in biological washing powders), 1,2-benzisothiazol, 2-octyl-2H-isothiazol-3, 5-chloro-2-methyl-4-iso-thiazolin-3-one, 2-methyl-2H-isothiazol-3-one. Most of these substances are classified as 'hazardous' and as 'biocides'; that is, in the same category as pesticides; they damage living organisms. Some detergents also contain phenols and ammonia, both toxic, and artificial fragrances ('parfum'), of which more later. Cleaning chemicals especially endanger your lungs.[3] And children are most at risk.[4]

But we have to get things clean! Well, yes, but what do we mean by 'clean'? We tend to think 'clean' means free of all micro-organisms, all bacteria. But only an operating theatre needs to be that sterile; our kids' immune systems, and our own, do need to encounter some bugs in order to mature and function properly. A sterile kitchen is one that encourages allergies; there really is such a thing as too much hygiene! Not all bugs are unfriendly, and some are vital. I would ditch the anti-bacterial wipes and sprays completely, and replace all the other products as follows.

Washing-up Liquid

Use a safe, 'green' brand such as Ecover or, even better, Suma's Ecoleaf. These are not perfect, but they're an awful lot better than the standard ones.

Laundry Powder

The same applies to your laundry powder, with which you can, by the way, use about a quarter of the recommended amounts, even with Suma, Ecover or Allavare, as recommended in chapter 3. Less is more. (Powder is better than liquid, as a rule; less likely to make the washing machine mouldy.) Standard laundry products are associated with eczema in children, in my experience. And that's just an obvious, immediate effect. The Soil Association recommend Greenscents products for washing up, surface cleaners, laundry and more. Their recommendation means it will be truly organic.

Surface Cleaning

You can just use a damp cloth or bicarbonate of soda (sodium bicarbonate), a simple, alkaline white powder (yes, it's baking powder), which also cleans ovens, grills, fridges – and teeth! It can be used to deodorise a smelly fridge too (comes in handy if you've left teenagers unattended for a weekend).

Drain Cleaning

First, do some prevention: don't let grease or vegetable bits go down the sink. Second, pour boiling water down there or clean drains with a mixture of sodium bicarbonate, vinegar and ordinary salt. It fizzes and it cleans.

Windows

Many people use vinegar, which does work, but I prefer my house not to smell like a chippy, so I just use warm water. It also works. If necessary, add a tiny amount of (eco-friendly) washing up liquid to the warm water.

Furniture

You can use beeswax polish. Removing stains from carpets and soft furnishings is trickier – I deal with it below in the 'Living Room' section.

Pots and Pans

What are you cooking your food in? Aluminium pans can be problematic, because aluminium is a toxic metal, implicated in Alzheimer's Disease, autism and breast cancer.[5] But surely the aluminium doesn't get into the food? Well, that depends on what you cook in it. Boiling an egg or some rice or pasta is fine. But anything acid will leach the metal out of the pan into your food (that's just basic chemistry), so tomato sauce, rhubarb, apples, pears, plums or anything with lemon juice in should never be cooked in an aluminium pan. If you are diabetic, I would avoid cooking such foods in stainless steel pans too, because stainless steel is 14 per cent nickel, and nickel is implicated in abnormal sugar metabolism,[6] so it may make diabetes worse.[7]

Non-stick pans are now known to be a real hazard; what makes them non-stick is Teflon or similar substances, which contain PFAs, perfluoroalkyl and polyfluoroalkyl substances. Remember the 'fluoro' in there; it's fluoride and it contributes mightily to the toxicity of these substances. The PFAs accumulate in all our organs and are linked with cancer, polycystic ovary syndrome, thyroid problems, heart disease, liver damage, premature birth and low birth weight and doubtless many more diseases to be uncovered. As soon as one of these substances is banned, another pops up, allegedly safer – till it turns out not to be, as we saw in chapter 3.

The Alternatives

Old-fashioned cast-iron pots are very safe (unless you have the rare inherited condition haemochromatosis) but they are heavy, so make sure you get one with two handles, for easier lifting. Same with Le Creuset pots, but do NOT get their new, non-stick versions, just the original enamel-lined ones. I know they are terribly expensive, but you only need one, and now you can wash it in safe, non-toxic washing-up liquid it will last for decades. But you do need to stir; they are not naturally non-stick. However, in Mongolia they cook in cast-iron pots and never wash the pot; they just wipe it out at the end of each meal. This eventually builds up a natural non-stick coating.[8] Glass pans are fine; borosilicate glass is designed to cope with high oven temperatures. Ceramic pans are fine too, and if you really want non-stick then there are safe, PFAs-free versions now, made by GreenPan or by GreenLife pans, which use sand and, believe it or not, diamonds, to make a safe non-stick surface. They are not cheap either, but it's worth saving up for one. Just don't fry at very high temperatures in them, because that will eventually erode the surface of any pan.

Food Containers and Wrappings

Silver foil is not silver, it's aluminium. It's ok to wrap your sandwiches in, but you don't want it in contact with anything acid (as above), so, if you are cooking meat or fish in the oven and you've squeezed lemon juice on it, please don't have foil touching the food. It's ok to use it as a lid across the top of the pot, so long as it's not in direct contact with the food. The simplest thing is just to use a pot with a lid if you're cooking in the oven.

With regard to wrapping/storing food, please don't use clingfilm or any other kind of plastic wrap. This is about a set of toxic hazards discussed in chapter 3: phthalates. These unpronounceable chemicals are plasticisers used to make plastics soft and flexible. They are endocrine disruptors, implicated in cancers of the male and female reproductive system, menstrual disturbances, fertility problems and possibly polycystic ovary syndrome (PCOS). They may also damage the thyroid gland.[9] The softer the plastic, the greater the amount of phthalates (and bisphenol A and other toxins) that get into the food. So, clingfilm is the worst, whereas storing food in a hard, solid plastic box in the fridge or freezer is much less of a concern. The lower the temperature and the harder the plastic, the less transfer of toxic plastics to the food, and thence to your body. (This is why you should never drink water from plastic bottles, especially if they are warm. Use glass.) You can wrap food in old-fashioned paper bags for a packed lunch ('If You Care' do packs of brown paper bags) and, at home, keep food in ceramic dishes in the fridge. These days you can get glass or ceramic boxes with plastic, wooden or bamboo lids. Cheese will keep fine in a butter dish; you really don't want it wrapped in soft plastic.

Unfortunately, some food or drink you buy may already be plastic wrapped. Not just food in plastic packaging, but milk or plant milks in plastic cartons. What's the carton lined with? Is it plastic? Does it tell you on the outside of the carton? Just one more thing to be aware of and investigate. And what about food in plastic wrapping that you put in the microwave oven? I would never recommend microwaving anyway, for the reasons explained in chapter 6, but an additional reason is that the high temperature in the microwave (or any oven) will release phthalates and other toxic plastic chemicals into your food. Plastics are as toxic for us as they are for oceans and wildlife; let's cut down on our use of them, to benefit our own health and that of the whole planet.

Your Kitchen Tap

What's coming out of it? Just water, right? Sorry, no. It's water plus a whole lot of things that shouldn't be in there. Firstly, **chlorine**, added by the water companies to remove pathogenic bacteria. As we've seen, chlorine is toxic and has been linked with asthma (from chlorinated swimming pools), colon cancer, suppression of thyroid hormone production and other problems. This isn't actually necessary; the Dutch disinfect their water quite safely using a combination of physical filters and ultra-violet light, as we learnt in chapter 3.

Then there is **fluoride**. Fluoride has been added to the water supply in Birmingham since 1964, and in my practice I have certainly seen a lot of bone-damaged and brain-damaged children from Birmingham with shockingly high levels of fluoride in their urine (again, see chapter 3 for more on this).

Then there are the substances that get into our water unintentionally, and that the water companies have no effective systems for removing. For example, every drug taken by us humans, whether prescribed, over-the-counter or illegal, is excreted in the urine and finds its way into the water table, the rivers,[10] and eventually into our drinking (and bathing) water. Then there are the antibiotics and other drugs given routinely to (non-organic) farm animals; the animals pee on the fields and the drug residues leach through the soil into the reservoirs and finally into us. Furthermore, herbicides, fungicides, insecticides and pesticides sprayed on the land run off into the water table and also find their way into our water.[11]

If you don't want to be drinking all this junk, you need to invest in a good-quality water filter. If you are renting, you'll need to get a counter-top version, but try to make sure that the water is filtering into a glass jug rather than a plastic one. If you own your home, it is worth getting a plumbed-in water filter. Then you'll be using filtered water not only for drinking but also for cooking, rinsing vegetables and fruit, and so on. If you can afford it, the ideal plumbed-in filter is a whole-house water filter, so you are bathing in safe water as well as drinking safe water. You'll notice that that faint smell of chlorine is gone – or you'll notice it for the first time staying in someone else's place. Some people notice that they no longer get itchy after a hot bath.

It is hard to recommend a particular water filter as there are so many on the market these days, but your main criteria should be: (a) that the company has been making water filters for several years (so they haven't just jumped on the bandwagon) and (b) that when you ask them exactly which toxins does this filter remove, and how, they can give you a clear, detailed, referenced, written answer. Check that it can remove halogens (that includes chlorine and fluoride), heavy metals, pesticide residues and drug residues. Take your time; it's a big deal. But it's worth it.

In the Bathroom

Mould

Is there any **mould**? Black mould can accumulate in areas that are perpetually damp (in kitchens as well as bathrooms) and although mould is 'natural', in the sense that it is a living organism (a fungus, in fact), it produces waste products called mycotoxins, which are as dangerous to us as any synthetic chemical and implicated in all sorts of illnesses from allergy and anaphylaxis to chronic fatigue and cancer. Prevention is better than cure (always); keep windows and doors open, so air can circulate, and keep the bathroom warm (even with windows open), to minimise dampness and thus discourage growth of mould. Moulds don't grow in hot, dry countries.

Clean off any visible mould with **borax** (from www.baldwins.co.uk) or a paste made at home from baking soda (again!) and water. If you suffer from asthma or arthritis the mould may be aggravating it; get someone else to clean it off for you, so you don't make yourself worse. Mould spores (and house dust mites) can be caught and removed from the air by a HEPA filter (high-efficiency particulate air filter), but you probably want to install this in the bedroom rather than the bathroom, as you spend one third of your life in the bedroom.

Air Fresheners

They do not really 'freshen' the air, they pollute it with poisons including formaldehyde, naphthalene, para-dichlorobenzene, toluene, benzene, xylene, styrene, phthalates (again) and more. We inhale these chemicals every time we spray; so do our kids, and so do our pets. Many of them are implicated in cancer and endocrine/reproductive disease.[12] A good question to ask is: why does the air in your house need 'freshening' anyway? Empty the bins and open the windows.

If you still want a nice smell, use essential oils such as lavender, lemongrass, orange flower, jasmine, geranium, bergamot, rose or frankincense. Just put them in a little ceramic burner above a tealight candle, ideally a beeswax candle rather than a standard petrochemical one. But certainly don't use scented candles – they are full of the same nasties. Ditto the plug-in versions. For beeswax candles, to ensure that they are completely organic and that the bees are looked after in a humane and ecologically sound way, the Soil Association recommend two brands, Skär Organics and Sacred and Wild.

Personal Care Products

This is a misnomer as most people's bathroom cabinets are full of petrochemical products that do not in fact care for the body, but rather damage it. I call them Personal Scare products. Synthetic soap and shampoo can be replaced by natural versions such as those made by Suma, Avalon Organics, Dr Bronner's or Urtekram. The Soil Association recommend Odylique's range of shampoos and conditioners, all certified by COSMOS (see below). Compare ingredients lists, as they do change sometimes. Moisturiser, usually full of toxic petrochemicals that are absorbed into the body, can be replaced by safe options like those made by Sukin, Weleda or Green People – or you can just use coconut oil or shea butter. You'll find you need less moisturiser anyway if you change to natural soap and filter the chlorine out of your water.

When Is Organic Not Organic?

If you choose personal care products labelled 'organic', you should be safe, right? Well, so I thought, until I was enlightened by Paige Tracey of the Soil Association. Paige is in charge of the organic certification of their 'non-food' products, and that includes 'beauty' products. I was shocked to learn from her that it is perfectly legal in the UK to label a 'beauty' or 'well-being' product as organic if it contains only one per cent organic ingredients! Unlike with food, regulation is virtually non-existent. And yet whatever you put on your skin will be absorbed into your body as surely as if you had eaten it. The good news, though, is that the Soil Association has now teamed up with other organisations to form COSMOS, which certifies truly organic cosmetic products. Their standards, like those of GOTS for textiles (see chapter 3), are really high. There is a long list of unpleasant toxic compounds, which the Soil Association and COSMOS will not permit in the products they certify but which may well be found in other products hanging around on shop shelves cheekily calling themselves 'organic'. So, look out for the COSMOS label and do have a good look at the Soil Association's 'Health and Beauty' pages; they have some excellent recommendations, far more than I have space to share here.

Make-up

With make-up and make-up remover it's harder, but still possible, to find safer brands like Pure Mineral from Elemental Beauty. Uoga Uoga is a COSMOS-certified make-up brand recommended by the Soil Association. But I would seriously consider ditching make-up altogether; after all, if your face is covered in foundation, whether mineral or not, the sunlight cannot get through to your skin to make vitamin D. Nail varnish is harder still, but the key thing is to apply it outdoors, so you are not inhaling so much of the toxic fumes; once it's dried on it is no longer a problem. Same with nail-varnish remover.

Hair Dye

These are toxic; they have been linked with bladder cancer and breast cancer,[13] but there are a few safer versions, such as pure, natural henna and a brand called It's Pure. You don't want toxic hair dyes touching your scalp, because they'll be absorbed into your bloodstream. 'Dip-dyeing' is ok, though, because then the dye only goes on the ends of your hair, not into your body. Hair sprays, perming lotions and straightening lotions are similarly full of lethal substances that have been linked with cancers of the womb, ovary and breast.[14] So, hairdressers are particularly at risk.

Bubble Bath

You can replace bubble bath with any combination of the essential oils in the Air Fresheners section on page 172; they provide lovely smells, but it has to be admitted that they don't make bubbles.

Sunscreen

These usually contains titanium dioxide and other nasties, which get into our bodies through our skin,[15] and some dermatologists fear that it's actually sunscreen, rather than sunshine, that is causing the rising incidence of skin cancer.[16] Conventional sunscreens can be replaced by those made by Odylique, Sweet Bee Organics or Badger; at time of writing their ingredients lists are all ok. Or just cover up with white cotton clothing. (Information on how to tan slowly and safely is in *SAITT*, on pages 103–106.)

Deodorants

Deodorants are a bit of a minefield. Most contain parabens and aluminium, both of which are toxic, and aluminium has been linked with Alzheimer's disease, autism and breast cancer.[17] There are some alternatives on the market that claim to be safe, but if you look closely you'll see that the ingredients list often includes 'natural rock alum'. It's still aluminium! I think if we wash regularly, we shouldn't actually need deodorant; it's time to reacclimatise to the smell of fresh, healthy, natural human sweat. It only smells bad if it's old or if it's the sweat of fear. And we certainly don't want antiperspirants because sweating is one of the body's ways of detoxing; it makes little sense to prevent that. Secondary schools need to stop their insistence on deodorants in the sports changing room; these toxins being sprayed around at close quarters are doing the kids no good and making the chemically sensitive kids quite ill. There are some genuinely organic brands, though; the Soil Association recommend Haoma.

Perfume

This is another minefield, and not only perfume in its own right, but 'parfum' or 'fragrance' as an (unspecified) ingredient of all the above 'personal care' products (and many kitchen cleaning products). Modern commercial perfume is not made of flower essences, it's made of petrochemicals such as benzene, toluene, parabens, phthalates and synthetic musk. Most of these ingredients are known carcinogens – and that's just those that are displayed on the label – and they are absorbed through our skin straight into the body. The manufacturers are not required by law to disclose every ingredient and the average bottle of perfume contains fourteen unlisted ingredients![18] The solution is just to use natural, organic essential oils, as I detail in Air Fresheners on page 172. No, they won't last all day because they are natural, so the body knows how to biodegrade them. Anything that lasts all day is synthetic and worrying.

Dental Care

Your toothpaste probably contains fluoride and your dentist has probably told you that fluoride is good, even essential, for your teeth. I beg to differ, as there is much evidence that fluoride does more harm than good (see chapter 3). I would advise a fluoride-free toothpaste such as those made by Green People. Georganics and Organically Epic are other options, recommended by the Soil Association. Even your dental floss may be a source of problems; that nice, free-sliding, waxy texture is due to PFAs, the toxins mentioned above in connection with non-stick pans. You can get a safe dental floss made of bamboo or silk from Woo Bamboo; it comes from the US but is sold in many health food shops in the UK. Also, check your mouthwash if you use one; a lot of brands have fluoride in now. We shouldn't swallow this! Periobrite is a safe, fluoride-free brand, though you might find it cheaper to ask a herbalist to make one up for you from scratch.

Menstrual Products

Pads and tampons may cause allergic reactions[19] and may contain dioxins, pesticides, bleach (chlorine) and other nasties; it is safest to get a brand made from 100 per cent organic cotton, such as Natracare (www.natracare.com); and also check out the Campaign for Safe Cosmetics (www.safecosmetics.org). Much more on menstrual products – and nappies (diapers) – in chapter 3.

Head Lice

If you have children of primary-school age, your bathroom cabinets may contain products to get rid of head lice and nits (the eggs of lice) from their hair. These are toxic insecticides and you don't want to be putting them on your child's scalp. Luckily, there is an alternative that is not only safe and chemical-free, but has also been shown to be more effective.[20] Bug Buster kits can be ordered from the NHS-approved charity Community Hygiene Concern, via www.chc.org.

Fleas

Similarly, to prevent pet fleas, you may have flea collars (they're impregnated with insecticides) on your pets, or maybe you let the vet put insecticides on them every few months. Don't. It's hazardous for the pets, and for the children (and adults) who stroke them. (Vets don't tend to use the term 'insecticide'. They'll just tell you the brand name of the latest one that's being promoted. But an insecticide it usually is.)

Instead, you can get powdered neem leaf from any good herbal supplier and rub it into the cat or dog's fur. All over. It turns your animal rather green for a day or two, but it kills or at least repels the fleas, and when the animal licks it off it acts as a natural dewormer too. It's a traditional Indian herbal remedy from the neem tree, and safer all round. It's better for prevention than cure, though, like most natural remedies; use it early in spring a few times, before the 'flea season' gets going! You can also use diatomaceous earth,[21] which is a form of silica, to put on the cat or dog, or on the floor if you're unfortunate enough to get fleas in the carpet. It simply dries the insects out, so they die from desiccation, but it's not poisonous. However – and this is an important warning – you need to put a mask on when applying it, especially if you're asthmatic, because it's a fine powder and you don't want to inhale it. You vacuum it up after a couple of days.

There are also some flea-killing essential oils, which may be safe on dogs, but they're NOT safe on cats. For prevention of fleas, the vet can give your pet an injection of Program every six months. It's not an insecticide; it merely sterilises the fleas and doesn't harm you or your pet. Program used to be available as a capsule, the contents of which you'd put in your pet's food, but annoyingly it is now only available as an injection from the vet.

In the Bedroom

Mattresses

Most standard mattresses contain all sorts of synthetic chemicals including VOCs.[22] These are volatile organic compounds, but this doesn't mean 'organic' in the sense of your nice pesticide-free veg; it's a chemical term meaning that the molecule contains carbon. These chemicals 'outgas' while you are sleeping and include toxins such as chloromethane, acetone, propranolol and toluene. Mattresses also contain toxic flame-retardants such as polybrominated biphenyls (PBBs – see chapter 3). They get into you both by inhalation and via the skin. If your mattress is older than two years, it's probably finished 'outgassing', so don't panic. But if you are thinking of getting a new mattress, please try to get an organic one. The Natural Mat and Abaca Organic are two reliable companies, and Hypnos organic mattresses are recommended by the Soil Association. A safe mattress is essential for all of us and especially for children.

Your Wardrobe

Some people use moth balls in their wardrobes or chest of drawers, but these contain para-dichlorobenzene, a toxic insecticide.[23] It was the commonest toxin I found when testing sick patients in my practice. You can kill and prevent moths just as easily with lavender oil or a combination of lavender and neem provided in the safe moth spray from Greenfibres of Totnes.

Dry Cleaning

Your clothes are hanging up in your bedroom – but they present no hazard, surely? Well, normally not, but they do if you've just had them dry cleaned. Dry-cleaning fluids contain trichloroethylene and tetrachloroethylene, which are some of the most carcinogenic substances known, according to IARC, the International Agency for Research on Cancer.[24] So, if you must go to the dry cleaners, do it in summer, when you can hang the dry-cleaned clothes out on the line for few days to 'outgas' before bringing them back into your house.

In the Living Room, Hall, Landing – Everywhere!

Floors

First things first: take your shoes off when you come in! There's particulate matter (PM) from car exhaust fumes on the pavement, so it's on the soles of your shoes. Leave them near the front door; you don't want that PM pollution on your floors, especially if you have babies crawling around.

Even without PM pollution from outdoors, your carpet is probably impregnated with the same sort of toxins as are found in mattresses. If you can, it's better to have wooden floors (real wood rather than laminate) and washable rugs. Organic carpets are hard to come by and are not dyed, so they tend to be sheep coloured, which means that they show the dirt. Again, if your carpet is over two years old, don't worry, it has probably stopped outgassing. But if you are thinking of buying a new one, consider alternative, non-toxic floorings, such as organic wool rugs from www.nuloom.com, https://secondnatureonline.co.uk or www.naturalrugstore.co.uk and newer flooring materials such as cork, coir (coconut fibre), sisal, seagrass and bamboo.

Soft Furnishings

Many of these companies, and www.homescapesonline.com and www.ecosofa.co.uk, also do organic soft furnishings, such as sofas. Why do you need that? Because conventional sofas, for the first couple of years, outgas similar problematic chemicals, including the fire-retardant PBBs. These are only needed (and required by law) because synthetic soft furnishings are highly flammable. Whereas natural materials like wool and cotton are naturally flame-resistant. But if you get wool or cotton, ensure it's organic, otherwise it may be full of insecticides. What a complicated world we live in!

Also check out www.ecofurnitureuk.com, who make wooden sofa bases and bed bases and can arrange for them to be upholstered with natural fibres.

Cleaning

For removing **stains** from existing carpets and sofas, here's what Pat Thomas suggests in her book, *Cleaning Yourself to Death*: add half a cup of borax to one litre of warm water. Use a stiff bristle brush for carpets and a softer one like an old toothbrush for the sofa. Vacuum when dry. You can steam clean carpets with nothing but water, omitting the chemicals. And, of course, you can take your shoes off whenever you come in, to minimise the cleaning needed.

Decorating

How about decorating? Most paints are petrochemical-based and affect some people quite badly. Even if you don't react symptomatically, you might want to know that professional painters have an increased risk of cancer.[25] The good news is that there are now plenty of paints that are water-based and very safe, from companies such as Graphenstone, Ecos and Auro. The unpleasant solvents in glues and DIY products do not, to my knowledge, have safe alternatives yet, but just do the DIY in spring/summer and keep the windows open. Once it's dried you don't have to worry, so if you are very chemically sensitive you may need to go away for a couple of days while someone else does the DIY.

Electromagnetic Radiation

Lastly, there is another hazard in your home that you may not have thought about. You can't see it and you can't smell it, but in recent years you may have become mightily dependent on the devices that emit it. It's electromagnetic radiation (EMR), and it's coming out of your mobile phone, your cordless landline (and the DECT base that charges it), your wi-fi router, your laptop, your microwave oven, your smart meter if you have one (just say 'No!') and – horror – your baby monitor.

EMR is especially dangerous to children, and to the egg and sperm that will one day produce children. Don't keep your phone in your pocket when it's on or you'll be irradiating your testes or ovaries and messing with the DNA of your future offspring. That's as well as endangering your own health. Keep the phone on flight mode – or actually off – whenever possible. Put the laptop on a table, not your lap, especially if you are or might be pregnant. Turn the wi-fi off at night and whenever you are not using it. You can access the internet safely by using an ethernet cable. There are several companies now making stuff to protect you from EMR, and three of the best are Conscious Spaces, Beneficial Environments and Safe Living Technologies. There is much more about how to reduce, avoid and mitigate your EMR exposure in chapter 6.

CONCLUSION

OUR BODIES, OUR EARTH

In writing this book, I've encountered many wonderful scientists and campaigners. Some are aware of the danger of pesticides and are trying to save us from that. Others are raising the alarm about what fluoride is doing to us or the risks of heavy metal contamination. Still others are warning about the hazards that plastics pose to the planet and to all life upon it. Some are trying to stop the dumping of sewage into our water, some are campaigning for air that is safe for our children to breathe. Some have been researching and writing for decades about the dangers of nuclear power, and others about the greatly underestimated risks that mobile phones, mobile-phone masts, microwaves and wi-fi pose to us and to wildlife. A few scientists have actually noticed and documented the vast increase in cancer, neurodegenerative disease and other illnesses that is resulting from all of this. And this is not just among humans; experienced vets are noticing that our dogs are not living as long as they used to.

Each of these scientists and campaigners is doing a vital job. Each is holding one piece of the puzzle. It may be impossible, intellectually and emotionally, for anyone to hold The Whole Picture, but something like that is what I've attempted, perhaps rashly, to do in this book. It has felt, at times, like living in what Douglas Adams called the Total Perspective Vortex. Yet it's certainly not complete; there are numerous topics I haven't had space to cover, such as noise pollution, light pollution or occupational illness from exposure to specific chemicals.

So how do you, dear reader, choose what to do? Take it slowly. The information is yours, now, to do with as you will. Every little helps and each change makes a difference. You don't need to make all the changes at once! Even with a growing awareness of the overview, you will probably feel drawn to one particular issue more than another. For yourself, the first steps are eating organic, filtering your water, moderating/mitigating your use of mobile-phone technology and going through your home with a fine-toothed comb and chapter 7 in hand. In terms of campaigning, go where your passion takes you. Pretty well any campaign you might be inspired to join is mentioned in one of the first six chapters.

The Power in You

This is about reclaiming control over our own health. I have to admit, I don't particularly like thinking of myself as a 'consumer' – the word seems to reduce a human being to just a mouth, endlessly wanting STUFF. But consumer power is real: if we can overcome our shopping addiction and stop buying all these unnecessary toxic products, manufacturers will stop making them. If we support the alternative, safe, natural products, those alternatives will thrive and so will we. In the end it's about breaking the 'tyranny of convenience', and creating new habits, especially in our homes, so home can become again the sanctuary it is meant to be.

Most challengingly, when we find ourselves asking the inevitable question 'But surely they wouldn't allow all this stuff to be sold if it was dangerous?' we need to face up to the answer: yes, they would, and they do. There is no 'they' looking after us; companies are just looking after their profits, while governments look the other way. It's up to us.

But where is the medical profession in all this? Shouldn't they – we – be on the frontline of the battle for human health? It has struck me that, of the books I've read about the devastating effects of environmental pollution on our health, most have been written by investigative journalists, not medics.[1] There are campaigns to save the whales, the hedgehogs, the bats, the birds, the beetles, tigers, rhinos and rainforests – quite right too. But there is no campaign that I know of to Save the Humans. I guess we imagine that the issue of human health is 'covered' by the existence of doctors, hospitals, the NHS – God bless. But they won't do it for us. They just pick up the pieces. But our species, homo not-very-sapiens, is endangered.

When I ask GPs and other fellow medics what they think are the main environmental determinants of disease and death, they say cigarette smoking and excess alcohol. Those are very important indeed, but not environmental in the sense I mean it in this book. Some of the more aware doctors may add that iatrogenic illness, illness caused by medical treatment, is the fifth leading cause of death in the world.[2] This is mostly due to adverse drug reactions, or ADRs. Perhaps I should have included them in this book; drugs as human poisons. After all, I did mention what those drugs are doing to the fish in our rivers! But space is limited.

Overall, the attitude of the medical profession at large is one of fatalism: 'Doctor, why has this happened to me? To my body?' 'Oh, it's just bad luck.' That is an astonishingly common response my patients have had from their GPs or hospital consultants, and it's remarkably unscientific. Science is supposed to be all about cause and effect. Yet we are not trained, in medical school, to wonder about causes, and thus prevention, of illness.

This fatalism has filtered through to the general public. So, when someone we love becomes seriously ill, what do we do with the inevitable sadness, despair or rage that follows? We don't ask why, but we channel our compassion and natural desire to help, to *do something*, into the outlets our society provides. We wear a pink ribbon, run marathons to raise money, or wear a hat on Wear a Hat Day. I salute the love and caring that are the source of these activities, but I worry. I worry that the money raised goes to charities that simply fund the research of the drug industry, which is looking for futile but profitable 'magic bullets', not at causes. I worry that wearing a pink ribbon does not prevent breast cancer, the causes of which we have seen in this book. And I worry that Wear a Hat Day will not prevent or cure a single brain tumour. But the people in the ads look incredibly cheerful; ecstatic, in fact. And the hats are very cool. I haven't been able to discover when Wear a Hat Day began, but I'll bet it was pretty recent. Ten years ago, I knew nobody with a brain tumour. Now, sadly, I know (or know of) many. Wear a Hat Day is one response to this rapidly increasing incidence. This book is another.

All the world's great spiritual traditions tell us that we are one with nature, with each other, with all beings. From Buddhism in the East to the Native American wisdom of the West, that is the message. The great Vietnamese Buddhist teacher Thích Nhất Hạnh called it 'interbeing'. We are not separate. If we attempt to separate ourselves, disaster follows. If we get hooked on money and power and 'stuff', we lose touch with our mother the earth; we lose the plot. As the Native American botanist Robin Wall Kimmerer puts it:

'All flourishing is mutual. We need acts of restoration, not only for polluted waters and degraded lands, but also for our relationship to the world.'[3]

When we finally realise that the decline in our loved ones' health is coming from the self-same causes as the forest fires on the other side of the globe, the same causes as the melting Arctic ice and the drowning tropical islands, the same causes as the missing dawn chorus and the mysteriously withering trees in our own local park – then perhaps we will see that it is all one fight: our right to a healthy life along with that of all our fellow beings on this planet. Healing our bodies and repairing the earth are one and the same project.

APPENDIX I

IT'S ENVIRON-MENTAL! BODY, BRAIN AND MIND

Mental illness – there's a lot of it about. In fact, it deserves a whole book in its own right – but this appendix is intended as a short summary of the most important ways in which pollution is damaging our brains and therefore our minds.

Of course, psychological distress is multifactorial; there are many causes. Social and economic conditions, traumatic experiences, lack of love, genetic tendencies, nutritional factors and environmental factors all play a part. So, environmental pollution is only one contributing factor, but it's an increasingly important one.[1] In terms of environmental toxicity, a person's environment can be toxic chemically, electromagnetically or psycho-spiritually, or all three, but it's the first two I'll be focusing on here.

The brain is part of the body, so any chemical or electromagnetic influences that upset the body will upset the brain too, and hence the mental state. In this, we have to include not just so-called mental illness but also neurodevelopmental disorders and learning disabilities, which are becoming more and more frequent among our children.

Reaching the Brain

Autism, ADHD, dyslexia and other increasingly common cognitive impairments have been linked with industrial chemicals, including mercury, lead, polychlorinated biphenyls, arsenic, toluene, fluoride, chlorpyrifos, tetrachloroethylene and many more.[2] Particulate matter (PM) from exhaust fumes is implicated in neurodegenerative diseases such as Alzheimer's occurring in young adults and even children.[3] PM pollution inhaled by pregnant women can damage their babies; one documented effect is sleep disruption in the children.[4] And it seems that poisonous car exhaust gases like nitrogen dioxide, as well as PM pollution, are contributing to the epidemic of Autistic Spectrum Disorders.[5]

Traffic fumes apparently increase the incidence of common mental disorders by up to 39 per cent! The studies that find this result do make sure to control for other factors, like poverty, which often go together with living on a busy main road; it really is the fumes that are having this effect.[6] And the incidence of depression and the risk of suicide are increased by PM air pollution too.[7]

Neurodegenerative diseases, as we've seen in earlier chapters, are at epidemic levels.

Ozone pollution is contributing to this epidemic – ozone from vehicle pollution damages the synapses in the brain.[8] Sufferers from dementia use mental health services too, as depression and anxiety are frequent problems for them; the more pollution they are exposed to, it seems, the more they need to use these services.[9]

Indoor pollution has a significant role; we know now that cleaning chemicals, personal care products, air freshener sprays, fumes out-gassing from new carpets, mattresses, sofas, MDF furniture and so on, are all petrochemicals. They are lipophilic (fat soluble), so they go right through our cell membranes (which are made largely of fat) and head straight for the fattiest organ in the body: the brain.

Mould is an especially nasty indoor pollutant, which seems to be implicated in mental illness as well as in cancer and CFS.[10] Information on how to remove and prevent it is in the section In the Bathroom on page 171, and I give more detail in my first book, *SAITT*, on pages 129–130. It's well worth checking out an article by Dr Mary Ackerley called 'Brain on Fire: The Role of Toxic Mold in Triggering Psychiatric Symptoms'.[11] Dr Ackerley is one of a growing band of 'integrative psychiatrists', who are looking at the role of pollution, nutrition and toxic microbes in triggering mental illnesses that have hitherto been regarded as solely psychological phenomena. They are talking increasingly about the role of neuroinflammation; see also a more recent article, 'Brains on Fire: Swollen Brains, Toxins and Neuroinflammation'.[12]

As well as air pollution, all the environmental toxins we have discussed in this book have a role in damaging the brain and thus affecting mental function, especially the pesticides in non-organic food, the fluoride currently in the water in some areas of the UK (and most areas of the US) and the heavy metals. The heavy metals most involved in damaging the brain are lead, aluminium and mercury. Aluminium is implicated in both autism and Alzheimer's, and the many and various ways that mercury damages the brain are overwhelmingly documented. In chapter 2 of this book, you will find information on how to avoid these toxic metals, and in *SAITT* you will find info on how to detox them; that is, how get them out of your system.

In treating any form of mental distress to which environmental toxins have contributed, we can't separate environmental factors from nutritional factors. This is because toxins are anti-nutrients, and nutrients are anti-toxins. For example: zinc and magnesium deficiency exacerbate disorders like ADHD, but heavy metals like mercury, nickel and cadmium push these good minerals out of the body. So nutritional deficiency and environmental contamination are often two sides of one coin.

Furthermore, the liver's detoxification enzymes have to work hard to get rid of toxins. These liver detox enzymes need vitamin C, all the B vitamins and many minerals as cofactors. So, pollution, by calling upon the detox enzymes to overwork, will deplete these good nutrients. Conversely, poor nutrition will exacerbate the damaging effects of pollution on the brain and body. The ecological medicine solution is to put the Good Stuff In (nutrition) and then take the Bad Stuff Out (detox). In *SAITT*, you will learn how to do both.

Lastly, we have seen the devastating impact that electromagnetic radiation can have on the brain. Causing brain tumours is just the most extreme outcome, and takes many years to manifest, but, well before that stage, both people who know they are electro-sensitive and many who don't can suffer all sorts of emotional and cognitive impacts from exposure to EMR. Protecting themselves as described in chapter 6 can make all the difference, but I won't pretend it's easy. For some people who are suffering with their mental health, it is hard to implement the necessary changes. That's where support comes in. They need a good friend, a caring partner, a parent, sibling or adult child to support them in making the changes. When that person is there, willing and able to help, we see significant clinical improvement.

APPENDIX II

IN YOUR BACKYARD

Sometimes, the pollution is all in one place, and the people who live there suffer most. Occasionally these events make the headlines, but never for very long.

Local Episodes of Poisoning the People for Profit

In South Cambridgeshire in the UK, residents of Hauxton, Harston and ten other villages have been getting ill. Breathing difficulties, numb tongues, fatigue and more. There's a site there on which pesticides and herbicides have been produced since the 1940s. The land is seriously contaminated with dozens of toxic chemicals. Around 2010, the local council sold the contaminated site to a housing developer that made only a token effort to clean it up – they dug up the contaminated ground and laid it out in rows for the toxic chemicals to evaporate. They should have done this under cover and then transported the toxic soil away in covered lorries to avoid polluting the air. Then they should have used the site for a tarmacked car park, if anything – certainly not for homes for humans.

A similar money-saving, inadequate clean-up happened in Corby in Northamptonshire, where the toxic chemical dust from an old steelworks ended up being distributed around the town in uncovered lorries, and at least sixteen babies were later born with serious limb deformities. This and some other comparable cases from the UK and around the world are mentioned in *SAITT* on pages 149–150, but I only know about the Cambridgeshire scandal because a patient of mine lives in one of the affected villages and members of their family became ill. I am not using my informant's name at their request because, as they wrote to me, 'the company bosses can be legally vindictive'. But you can find more info on the Hauxair campaign website: www.thestunthouse.com/hauxair.

A similar situation is unfolding now in the village of Somercotes in Derbyshire, where Amber Valley Borough Council plans to allow housing development on an old landfill site known to contain dioxins and other dangerous substances; it used to be a mining area. Local people protested, the council ignored them, the developers gave false reassurances; that's the pattern. The moment the developers started digging, two people in Birchwood Lane in Somercotes, right next to the site, were taken to hospital: one with symptoms resembling a stroke, another with apparent seizures. Enquiries locally uncovered weird skin rashes and an unexpected number of cancer cases, among dogs as well as people. I haven't been able to find a website devoted to this issue yet, but, if you're in south Derbyshire, do try to learn more.

The Grenfell Tower tragedy in London on 14 June 2017 is far better known. But, as well as the seventy-two people who lost their lives in the fire – which spread rapidly through the whole building because of the appalling, money-saving way it had been created – there is also the lesser-known tragedy of the young firefighters who attended the blaze and are now dying of cancer. At least a dozen have been diagnosed with either digestive cancers or leukaemia, and I suspect, sadly, that number will go up. The toxins they inhaled that night – despite their protective gear – are also the responsibility of whoever built that shoddy tower, again putting profits before people's lives.

In the US, there are countless similar examples. In the town of Anniston, Alabama, the river ran red; not blood, but contamination with PCBs, toxic chemicals like dioxins that have now been banned, but which last for years. Monsanto, the company responsible for this (and for the similar dioxin, Agent Orange, that defoliated South Vietnam) had been making toxins in Anniston since the 1920s. They finally had to pay compensation to residents after a court case that concluded in 2003. But the money can't bring back all those who died before their time.

Chloroprene is a chemical manufactured to make synthetic rubber. It had for over fifty years been manufactured by DuPont in the Pontchartrain works in Louisiana. The nearest town, Reserve, has the nickname 'Cancer Alley' – it has the highest cancer rate in the US. Chloroprene is a known carcinogen and those in the local community who have not yet died of cancer are still fighting for justice. DuPont recently sold the site, as it would be 'too expensive' to clean it up.

There are countless more examples, including the cancer deaths and birth deformities around the burning oil fields of Iraq and the explosions and oil spills such as Piper Alpha, Deepwater Horizon, Exxon Valdez and many more. Usually, it turns out, someone has cut corners to save money and/or someone was asleep at the wheel. But we all need to wake up and smell the poison; whether it's next door, down the street or on the other side of the globe; no pollutant remains local for long. It travels on the wind and rain, and reaches us eventually, unless we find out, protect and protest.

RESOURCES

Many references and some website addresses are given in the main text of the book, but there is always more to know. So, if you'd like more information about any of the topics covered in this book, and/or you want to become involved in campaigning to make a difference to our health and our planet's health, this section gives you details of organisations and websites that can help you find your area of interest and take action.

Chapter One: Earth I

Veg Boxes

All produce from Riverford – www.riverford.co.uk – is completely organic. They sell butter, cheese, eggs, meat and hummus, as well as fruit and veg, and you can order what you want each week. Almost all of their produce is grown in the UK or in mainland Europe, and you have the option to order a 'UK only' box, but when their produce is from further afield it is still seasonal and never airfreighted.

Pulses

Hodmedods – www.hodmedods.co.uk – is another wonderful company. It specialises in beans and pulses, many of which were traditionally grown in the UK and now are again, thanks to Hodmedods; they support farmers to grow these pulses, and also grains, regeneratively, by guaranteeing them a market. Farmers want to do the right thing, but they have to be able to make a living. Pulses are good for the soil, as we've seen, and they're also a great source of vegetable protein for humans. And buying them from Hodmedods means they're not being imported from the other side of the world.

Safe Wheat

Another excellent project is Wildfarmed – www.wildfarmed.co.uk – founded by the musician Andy Cato. His farms grow wheat without chemicals, using all the regenerative methods described in Down on the Farm in chapter 1, so if you buy their flour to make bread you know there will be no carcinogenic glyphosate in your sandwiches.

Further Organisations

Here is a list of some more excellent organisations that you should know about.

Agricology: www.agricology.co.uk. How to make farming wildlife-friendly – agroecology.

Biodynamic Association: www.biodynamic.org.uk. Biodynamic is like regen + organic + permaculture + more; based on anthroposophy, going since the 1920s.

ClientEarth: www.clientearth.org. An environmental charity who use the law to tackle companies and governments on environmental issues.

Compassion in World Farming: www.ciwf.org.uk. How to farm without cruelty to animals; a longstanding campaign group.

The Ethical Butcher: www.ethicalbutcher.co.uk. Supplier of ethically farmed meat.

Ethical Consumer: www.ethicalconsumer.org. Info on how to live ethically in many aspects of life.

Extinction Rebellion: www.extinctionrebellion.uk. They organise marches and protests about climate change.

FarmED: www.farm-ed.co.uk. A new centre for food and farm education, making the links between farm and food and health.

Farming and Wildlife Advisory Group: www.fwag.org.uk. Helping farmers transition to more nature-friendly methods

Food for Life: www.foodforlife.org.uk. A Soil Association project working to get healthy organic food into schools.

Friends of the Earth: www.friendsoftheearth.uk. The longstanding environmental campaign group.

Garden Organic: www.gardenorganic.co.uk. For help with organic gardening.

Greenpeace: www.greenpeace.org.uk. A wonderful organisation campaigning on many vital issues.

Groundswell: www.groundswellag.com. An annual conference on regenerative farming.
Incredible Edible Network: www.incredibleedible.org.uk. Helping communities to grow and share good food.
Landworkers' Alliance: www.landworkersalliance.org.uk. A union of farmers, foresters and growers supporting agroecological approaches and opposing the industrialisation of agriculture.
Natoora: www.natoora.com. An excellent organic food retailer.
Oxford Real Farming Conference: www.orfc.org.uk. The leading annual conference on truly regenerative farming.
Permaculture Association: www.permaculture.org.uk. How to do gardening in a nature-friendly way; organic and more.
Real Seeds: www.realseeds.co.uk. Vegetable seeds that are definitely not GMOs!
The Sustainable Food Trust: www.sustainablefoodtrust.org. A wonderful organisation committed to feeding everyone ethically, sustainably and healthily.
Unearthed: https://unearthed.greenpeace.org. Greenpeace's brave and important investigative journalism branch.
Whole Health Agriculture: www.wholehealthag.org. Helps livestock farms to reduce antibiotic use, farm healthily and use natural/alternative medicine where necessary.
Woodland Trust: www.woodlandtrust.org.uk. They do a lot on agroforestry these days.

Some Farms

Daylesford Organic: www.daylesford.com.
Gazegill Organics: www.gazegillorganics.co.uk.
Gothelney Farm: www.gothelneyfarmer.co.uk
Pipers Farm: www.pipersfarm.com.

And Three Good Films

Kiss the Ground: www.kissthegroundmovie.com. Excellent documentary on regenerative agriculture.
The Biggest Little Farm: www.apricotlanefarms.com. The biography of an American family becoming regenerative farmers, against all the odds.

Six Inches of Soil: www.sixinchesofsoil.org. Follows three young British farmers standing up against industrialised agriculture and learning to farm regeneratively. Informative and inspiring.

Magazine

Wicked Leeks: https: / / wickedleeks.riverford.co.uk. An informative magazine that you can order with your Riverford veg box.

Chapter Three: Water

Fluoride

There are campaigns to save us from the dangers of fluoride both in the UK and the US.

In the UK: **Fluoride-Free Alliance**, www.ukfffa.org.uk.
In the US: **Fluoride Action Network**, www.fluoridealert.org.

And see pages 273–278 of *SAITT* for an introduction to the halogens (the class of elements to which fluoride belongs).

Safe and Sustainable Textiles

There's lots of information in chapter 3, in the section called Let's Go Natural (see page 86), but here is some more.

If you are not into sewing yourself, Izzy (based in Bristol, UK) is one of the many amazing people making old textiles into new clothes. Check her out at: www.worntothreads.com.

In Switzerland, there is Ocean Safe (I know, Switzerland is landlocked – but they still care), which produces non-toxic, biodegradable, organic textiles as part of the 'circular textile economy': nothing wasted, and there is nothing that can't be recycled or reused. It's run by Manuel Schweizer and can be found at www.ocean safe.co. In Canada, check out Ocean Wise (www.ocean.org), who have produced a short but comprehensive report called 'Me, My Clothes and the Ocean'.

Chapter Four: Air

Here are the names of some of the impressive organisations who are working, in various ways, to make our air fit to breathe.

Campaign for Better Transport: www.bettertransport.org.uk. A well-established campaign group.
Clean Air in London: www.cleanair.london.
Clean School Air: www.cleanschoolair.com.
ClientEarth: www.clientearth.org. A wonderful environmental charity that uses the law to challenge companies that pollute our world and the governments who let them get away with it.
Cycling UK: www.cyclinguk.org.
Living Streets: www.livingstreets.org.uk.
Moms' Clean Air Force: www.momscleanairforce.org.
Mums for Lungs: www.mumsforlungs.org. An excellent campaigning group, who make great A5 leaflets you can offer to drivers who leave their engines running while they are stationary; they advise to smile and be pleasant, offer the leaflet and leave. I've tried it – it works!
Street Space: www.wearestreetspace.org.
Sustrans: www.sustrans.org.uk. Work to promote cycling and walking and other sustainable transport options.
Transport and Environment: www.transportenvironment.org. Campaigning for less polluting transport in Europe.
Transport for All: www.transportforall.org.uk. For disabled travellers – see their report called 'Pave the Way'.

Chapter Five: Fire I

Check out the following organisations campaigning against nuclear power.

CND Cymru: www.cndcymru.org. CND in Wales. CND is the Campaign for Nuclear Disarmament, founded in 1957 by Bertrand Russell and others.
Nuclear Free Local Authorities: www.nuclearpolicy.info.

PAWB: www.stop-wylfa.org. People Against Wylfa-B. Wylfa-B is a proposed nuclear facility on the Welsh island of Anglesey. PAWB also means 'everybody' in Welsh.
Save the Severn: www.save-the-severn.com.
STAND: www.nuclearsevernside.co.uk. Severnside Together Against Nuclear Development.

Chapter Six: Fire II

Protect and Protest!

About electromagnetic pollution: as well as protecting ourselves personally, we need to learn more, raise awareness and protect those we love and others further afield. There are an increasing number of professional and citizen groups getting informed and taking action. Here's a selection of the best.

Action Against 5G: www.actionagainst5g.org. They took a case to court with the support of the famous human rights lawyer Michael Mansfield.
Electrosensitivity UK: www.es-uk.info. Produce a regular newsletter and support ES/EHS sufferers.
EM Radiation Research Trust: www.radiationresearch.org. Supports ES sufferers. Lots of useful information.
Environmental Health Trust: www.ehtrust.org. Created by Dr Devra Davis to research environmental health hazards and safeguard human health through education and policy.
Europeans for Safe Connections: www.esc-info.eu.
International Appeal to Stop 5G on Earth and in Space: www.5gspaceappeal.org.
International Society of Doctors for the Environment: www.isde.org.
Microwave News: www.microwavenews.com. An excellent resource; it has been going for over forty years, run by Louis Slesin, PhD.
Physicians for Safe Technology: www.mdsafetech.org.
Physicians' Health Initiative for Radiation and Environment: www.phiremedical.org.

Powerwatch: www.powerwatch.org.uk. They have been going for a very long time, founded by electronic engineer and researcher Alasdair Philips; a superb source of information.
RF Info: www.rfinfo.co.uk. The RF stands for radio frequency. An excellent source for both info and campaigning.
Safe Schools Information Technology Alliance: www.ssita.org.uk. About the hazards of wi-fi in schools, and the safe alternatives.
Safe Tech International: www.safetechinternational.org. 'Uniting to Protect Life on Earth'.
Stop Smart Meters: www.stopsmartmeters.org.uk.
The International EMF Scientist Appeal: www.emfscientist.org.

Books

In addition to the books referenced in chapter 6, here are four others well worth checking out:

Overpowered by Martin Blank.
Disconnect by Devra Davis.
Radiation Nation by Daniel T. DeBaun and Ryan P. DeBaun.
*EMF*D* by Joseph Mercola.

Film

And here's a short film called *Remembering Nearfield* to watch:
www.vimeo.com/810958040.

Lastly, my website **www.drjennygoodman.com** has useful updates, including a list of recommended practitioners of ecological medicine, nutritional therapy and so on.

ACKNOWLEDGEMENTS

Thanks are due to the many people who have helped and encouraged me in the process of writing this book.

Firstly, I am grateful to all my wonderful colleagues in the British Society for Ecological Medicine, where I learnt – and learn – almost everything I know. In particular, Dr Rachel Nicoll has generously shared much valuable information, especially about heavy metal toxicity, and both she and Dr Shideh Pouria have been most supportive and encouraging of this challenging project. In researching organic and regenerative farming, I have received much useful information from Rebecca Hosking, Fred Price, Peter Greig, John Cherry, Russ Carrington and Fran Bailey, and I am grateful to Andrew Barr for pointing me towards the fascinating books of Graham Harvey on this topic, which led me on to the crucial work of Colin Tudge and others in this (pun intended) field.

In writing about the dangers of pesticides, I've been tremendously enlightened by Dr Stephanie Williamson and Josie Cohen of the Pesticide Action Network as well as Nick Mole and the director of PAN UK, Keith Tyrell. On the subject of safe/unsafe 'personal care products', Paige Tracey of the Soil Association has been a fount of vital and valuable facts. Amelia Twine of Sustainable Fashion Week and Emma Hague of Fibreshed have both been immensely helpful in the sphere of toxic versus sustainable clothing, a topic I knew far too little about before I started writing this book.

Graeme Munro-Hall gave me useful information about the latest legislation on mercury toxicity, and Joy Warren of the Fluoride-Free Alliance gave generously of her time discussing the hazards of fluoride and the campaigns to keep it out of the UK's drinking water.

On outdoor air pollution, I am grateful to Dr David Janner-Klausner for his generosity in giving of his time and considerable expertise, and to Alexander Massey for sharing his thoughts about the Low Traffic Neighbourhoods in Oxford. On the hazards of nuclear radiation, I am most grateful to Richard Bramhall of the Low Level Radiation Campaign for his support and for reading through the relevant chapter, and to the brilliant Professor Chris Busby for reading and checking this chapter too. In the hotly contested sphere of electromagnetic radiation, I am grateful to Karen Churchill and Amanda Kenton for keeping me in the loop about campaigns and court cases, and to the immensely knowledgeable Alasdair Philips of Powerwatch for generously taking the time, at short notice, to read and check the relevant chapter. Any errors that remain, in any chapter, are mine alone.

Special thanks to Leo Rutherford for long-time earth-based spiritual inspiration. And a big shout-out (is that what we say these days?) to George T. Maguire, who sends me zillions of relevant articles and manages for me what would otherwise be the utterly incomprehensible world of social media. George, you have achieved what many tried and failed: you've dragged me kicking and screaming into the twenty-first century. Couldn't have done it without you.

A huge thank you to Muna Reyal, my editor at Chelsea Green, who has been as patient, clear, skilful and lovely an editor as any author could dream of. And to the whole delightful CG team: thank you.

All my friends have been incredibly supportive of this project, and very understanding about my becoming uncharacteristically asocial, as I've spent a year or two being a hermit to get the book finished. I am deeply grateful to every one of you, but special mention must go to Jacqui Kashyap Lichtenstern, Aleda Erskine, Vivienne Cato, Shoshi Asheri, Suzette Clough, Rabbi Laura Janner-Klausner and my very special sister, Lynda Goodman. The sustained moral support has been so important. Thank you.

Lastly, and most of all, I am, as ever, profoundly grateful to my beloved husband, Dr Stuart Linke. For believing in me, for supporting and encouraging me, and for quietly getting on with my half of the domestic tasks that have been totally neglected throughout the more-than-a-year of writing fervour. Thank you so much. I do know how lucky I am.

NOTES

Introduction

1. Isabella Tree, *Wilding: The Return of Nature to a British Farm* (London: Picador, 2018), 147.
2. Jenny Goodman, *Staying Alive in Toxic Times: A Seasonal Guide to Lifelong Health* (London: Yellow Kite, 2020), 231–234.
3. Paul Clayton and Judith Rowbotham, 'How the Mid-Victorians Worked, Ate and Died', *International Journal of Environmental Research and Public Health* 6, no. 3 (2009): 1235–1253.
4. Philip J. Landrigan et al., 'The *Lancet* Commission on Pollution and Health', *The Lancet* 391, no. 10119 (2018): 462–512.
5. Adrian Goldberg and Ben Robinson, 'Skin Creams Containing Paraffin Linked to Fire Deaths', BBC News, 19 March 2017, https://www.bbc.co.uk/news/uk-39308748.

Chapter One

1. David R. Montgomery et al., 'Soil Health and Nutrient Density: Preliminary Comparison of Regenerative and Conventional Farming', *PeerJ* 10 (2022): e12848, https://doi.org/10.7717/peerj.12848.
2. Jordi Julvez et al., 'Early Life Multiple Exposures and Child Cognitive Function: A Multi-centric Birth Cohort Study in Six European Countries', *Environmental Pollution* 284 (2021): 117404, https://doi.org/10.1016/j.envpol.2021.117404.
3. Colin Tudge, *So Shall We Reap* (London: Allen Lane, 2003), 87.
4. Jane A. Plant, Nikolaos Voulvoulis and Kristín Vala Ragnarsdottir, eds., *Pollutants, Human Health and the Environment: A Risk Based Approach* (Chichester: Wiley-Blackwell, 2012), 182.
5. FAO, ITPS, GSBI, SCBD and EC, *State of Knowledge of Soil Biodiversity: Status, Challenges and Potentialities, Summary for Policymakers* (Rome, FAO, 2020), https://doi.org/10.4060/cb1929en.
6. Jørgen Stenersen, *Chemical Pesticides Mode of Action and Toxicology* (Boca Raton: CRC Press, 2004), https://doi.org/10.1201/9780203646830.

7. Sudisha Mukherjee and Rinkoo Devi Gupta, 'Organophosphorus Nerve Agents: Types, Toxicity, and Treatments', *Journal of Toxicology* 2020 (2020): 3007984, https://doi.org/10.1155/2020/3007984.

8. Alberto Ascherio et al., 'Pesticide Exposure and Risk for Parkinson's Disease', *Annals of Neurology* 60, no.2 (2006): 197–203, https://doi.org/10.1002/ana.20904.

9. Ioannis Zaganas et al., 'Linking Pesticide Exposure and Dementia: What is the Evidence?', *Toxicology* 307 (2013): 3–11.

10. Tesifón Parrón et al., 'Environmental Exposure to Pesticides and Cancer Risk in Multiple Human Organ Systems', *Toxicology Letters* 230, no. 2 (2014) 157–165, https://doi.org/10.1016/j.toxlet.2013.11.009.

11. Mengqi Wang et al., 'Atrazine Promotes Breast Cancer Development by Suppressing Immune Function and Upregulating MMP Expression', *Ecotoxicology and Environmental Safety* 253 (2023): 114691.

12. Deepika Kubsad et al., 'Assessment of Glyphosate Induced Epigenetic Transgenerational Inheritance of Pathologies and Sperm Epimutations: Generational Toxicology', *Scientific Reports* 9, no. 1 (2019): 6372.

13. Roy R. Gerona et al., 'Glyphosate Exposure In Early Pregnancy And Reduced Fetal Growth: A Prospective Observational Study Of High-Risk Pregnancies', *Environmental Health* 21, no. 1 (2022): 95, https://doi.org/10.1186/s12940-022-00906-3

14. Annette Abell, Erik Ernst and Jens Peter Bonde, 'High Sperm Density Among Members of an Organic Farmers' Association', *The Lancet* 343, no. 8911 (11 June 1994): 1498.

15. International Agency for Research on Cancer, *Q&A on Glyphosate* (Lyon: World Health Organization, 2016), https://www.iarc.who.int/wp-content/uploads/2018/11/QA_Glyphosate.pdf.

16. Robin Mesnage et al., 'Comparative Toxicogenomics of Glyphosate and Roundup Herbicides by Mammalian Stem Cell-Based Genotoxicity Assays and Molecular Profiling in Sprague-Dawley Rats', *Toxicological Sciences* 186, no. 1 (March 2022): 83–101, https://doi.org/10.1093/toxsci/kfab143.

17. Jørgen Stenersen, *Chemical Pesticides: Mode of Action and Toxicology* (Boca Raton: CRC Press, 2004), https://doi.org/10.1201/9780203646830.

18. Evanthia Diamanti-Kandarakis et al., 'Endocrine-Disrupting Chemicals: An Endocrine Society Scientific Statement', *Endocrine Reviews* 30, no. 4 (2009): 293–342, https://doi.org/10.1210/er.2009-0002.

19. Rebecca McKinlay, J.A. Plant, J.N.B. Bell and N. Voulvoulis, 'Endocrine Disrupting Pesticides: Implications for Risk Assessment', *Environment international* 34, no. 2 (2008): 168–183.

20. G. Van Maele-Fabry and J.L. Willems, 'Prostate Cancer Among Pesticide Applicators: A Meta-analysis', *International Archives of Occupational and Environmental Health* 77 no.8 (2004): 559–570.

21. Peter A. Clark, J. Chowdhury, B. Chan and N. Radigan, 'Chronic Kidney Disease in Nicaraguan Sugarcane Workers: A Historical, Medical, Environmental Analysis and Ethical Analysis', *Internet Journal of Third World Medicine* 12, no. 1 (2016).

22. Stephanie Seneff, *Toxic Legacy: How the Weedkiller Glyphosate is Destroying Our Health and the Environment* (White River Junction, VT: Chelsea Green, 2021).

23. Tom Blundell and Royal Commission on Environmental Pollution, *Crop Spraying and the Health of Residents and Bystanders* (London: Royal Commission on Environmental Pollution, 2005).

24. Neil Arya, 'Pesticides and Human Health: Why Public Health Officials Should Support a ban On Non-essential Residential Use', *Canadian Journal of Public Health* 96 (2005): 89–92.

25. Michael A.H. Bekken et al., 'Analysing Golf Course Pesticide Risk Across the US and Europe – The Importance of Regulatory Environment', *Science of the Total Environment* 874 (2023): 162498, https://doi.org/10.1016/j.scitotenv.2023.162498.

26. Marlaina S. Freisthler et al., 'Association Between Increasing Agricultural Use of 2,4-D and Population Biomarkers of Exposure: Findings from the National Health and Nutrition Examination Survey, 2001–2014', *Environmental Health* 21 (2022): 23, https://doi.org/10.1186/s12940-021-00815-x.

27. Anindita Mitra, Chandranath Chatterjee and Fatik B. Mandal, 'Synthetic Chemical Pesticides and Their Effects on Birds', *Research Journal of Environmental Toxicology* 5, no. 2 (2011): 81–96.

28. R. Mesnage et al., 'Impacts of Dietary Exposure to Pesticides on Faecal Microbiome Metabolism in Adult Twins', *Environmental Health: A Global Access Science Source* 21 no.1 (2022): 46, https://doi.org/10.1186/s12940-022-00860-0.

29. John Cherry, personal communication, 23 April 2023.

30. Graham Harvey, *We Want Real Food* (London: Robinson, 2008), 25.

31. Nader Rahimi Kakavandi et al., 'Maternal Dietary Nitrate Intake and Risk of Neural Tube Defects: A Systematic Review and Dose-response Meta-analysis', *Food and Chemical Toxicology* 118 (2018): 287–293.

32. E. Zohdi and M. Abbaspour, 'Harmful Algal Blooms (Red Tide): A Review of Causes, Impacts and Approaches to Monitoring and Prediction', *International Journal of Environmental Science and Technology.* 16 (2019): 1789–1806, https://doi.org/10.1007/s13762-018-2108-x.

33. Anna Bailey et al., 'Agricultural Practices Contributing to Aquatic Dead Zones', *Ecological and Practical Applications for Sustainable Agriculture* (2020): 373–393.

34. S. Joyce, 'The Dead Zones: Oxygen-Starved Coastal Waters', *Environmental Health Perspectives* 108, no. 3 (2000): A120–A125.

35. Sadie Costello et al., 'Parkinson's Disease and Residential Exposure to Maneb and Paraquat from Agricultural Applications in the Central Valley of California', *American Journal of Epidemiology* 169, no. 8 (2009): 919–926, https://doi.org/10.1093/aje/kwp006.

36. Emma Beswick, personal communication, 2022.

37. C.C. Lerro et al., 'Organophosphate Insecticide Use and Cancer Incidence Among Spouses of Pesticide Applicators in the Agricultural Health Study', *Occupational and Environmental Medicine* 72 (2015): 736–744.

38. Jerry Thompson, *Curing The Incurable: Beyond the Limits of Medicine – What Survivors of Major Illnesses Can Teach Us* (London: Hammersmith Health Books, 2020).

39. Lisa Volk-Draper et al., 'Paclitaxel Therapy Promotes Breast Cancer Metastasis in a TLR4-dependent Manner', *Cancer Research* 74, no. 19 (2014): 5421–5434; Laura G.M. Daenen et al., 'Chemotherapy Enhances Metastasis Formation via VEGFR-1–expressing Endothelial Cells', *Cancer Research* 71, no. 22 (2011): 6976–6985; Svetlana Gingis-Velitski et al., 'Host Response to Short-term, Single-agent Chemotherapy Induces Matrix Metalloproteinase-9 Expression and Accelerates Metastasis in Mice', *Cancer Research* 71, no. 22 (2011): 6986–6996; Serk In Park et al., 'Cyclophosphamide Creates a Receptive Microenvironment for Prostate Cancer Skeletal Metastasis', *Cancer Research* 72, no. 10 (2012): 2522–2532; Yi Seok Chang, Swati P. Jalgaonkar, Justin D. Middleton and Tsonwin Hai, 'Stress-inducible Gene Atf3 in the Noncancer Host Cells Contributes to Chemotherapy-exacerbated Breast Cancer Metastasis', *Proceedings of the National Academy of Sciences* 114, no. 34 (2017): E7159–E7168;

George S. Karagiannis et al., 'Neoadjuvant Chemotherapy Induces Breast Cancer Metastasis Through a TMEM-mediated Mechanism', *Science Translational Medicine* 9, no. 397 (2017): eaan0026; Dror Aleshekevitz et al., 'Macrophage-induced Lymphangiogenesis and Metastasis Following Paclitaxel Chemotherapy is Regulated by VEGFR3', *Cell Reports* 17, no. 5 (2016): 1344–1356.

40. Graeme Morgan, Robyn Ward and Michael Barton, 'The Contribution of Cytotoxic Chemotherapy to 5-year Survival in Adult Malignancies', *Clinical Oncology* 16, no. 8 (2004): 549–560.
41. Magdalena Czajka et al., 'Organophosphorus Pesticides can Influence the Development of Obesity and Type 2 Diabetes with Concomitant Metabolic Changes', *Environmental Research* 178 (2019): 108685, ISSN 0013–9351.
42. William Lana, personal communication, 2022.
43. Harvey, *We Want Real Food*, 219–220.
44. Montgomery et al., 'Soil Health and Nutrient Density', e12848.
45. Chloe MacLaren et al., 'Long-term Evidence for Ecological Intensification as a Pathway to Sustainable Agriculture', *Nature Sustainability* 5 (2022): 770–779.
46. Tudge, *So Shall We Reap*, 265.
47. Keith Tyrell, Director, Pesticide Action UK, personal communication, 31 January 2023.
48. Tyrell, personal communication. More info at: https://www.pan-uk.org/pesticide-poisoning.
49. Rachel Carson, *Silent Spring* (London: Penguin Random House, 2000).

Chapter Two

1. Jane A. Entwistle, Andrew S. Hursthouse, Paula A. Marinho Reis and Alex G. Stewart, 'Metalliferous Mine Dust: Human Health Impacts and the Potential Determinants of Disease in Mining Communities', *Current Pollution Reports* 5 (2019): 67–83.
2. Aristo Vojdani and Elroy Vojdani, 'The Role of Exposomes in the Pathophysiology of Autoimmune Diseases I: Toxic Chemicals and Food', *Pathophysiology* 28, no. 4 (2021): 513–543; G.M. Mujtba Hashmi and Munir H. Shah, 'Comparative Assessment of Essential and Toxic Metals in the Blood of Rheumatoid Arthritis Patients and Healthy Subjects', *Biological Trace Element Research* 146 (2012): 13–22; Robert L.

Siblerud and Eldon Kienholz, 'Evidence that Mercury from Silver Dental Fillings May Be an Etilological Factor in Multiple Sclerosis', *Science of the Total Environment* 142, no. 3 (1994): 191–205; S.V.S. Rana, 'Perspectives in Endocrine Toxicity of Heavy Metals – A Review', *Biological Trace Element Research* 160 (2014): 1–14, https://doi.org/10.1007/s12011-014-0023-7; Luísa Eça Guimarães, Britain Baker, Carlo Perricone and Yehuda Shoenfeld, 'Vaccines, Adjuvants and Autoimmunity', *Pharmacological Research* 100 (2015): 190–209, https://doi.org/10.1016/j.phrs.2015.08.003.

3. T. Coles at the Soil Association, personal communication, 14 July 2023.
4. Farhana Zahir, Shamim J. Rizwi, Soghra K. Haq and Rizwan H. Khan, 'Low Dose Mercury Toxicity and Human Health', *Environmental Toxicology and Pharmacology* 20, no. 2 (2005): 351–360.
5. Magnus Nylander, L. Friberg and B. Lind, 'Mercury Concentrations in the Human Brain and Kidneys in Relation to Exposure from Dental Amalgam Fillings', *Swedish Dental Journal* 11, no. 5 (1987): 179–187; Patrick Störtebecker, 'Mercury Poisoning from Dental Amalgam through a Direct Nose-brain Transport', *The Lancet* 333, no. 8648 (1989): 1207; M.J. Vimy and F.L. Lorscheider, 'Clinical Science: Intra-oral Air Mercury Released from Dental Amalgam', *Journal of Dental Research* 64, no. 8 (1985): 1069–1071, https://doi.org/10.1177/00220345850640080901.
6. Henrik Lichtenberg, 'Elimination of Symptoms by Removal of Dental Amalgam from mercury Poisoned Patients, As Compared with a Control Group of Average Patients', *Journal of Orthomolecular Medicine* 8 (1993): 145–145.
7. Dominik Nischwitz, *It's All in Your Mouth: Biological Dentistry and the Surprising Impact of Oral Health on Whole Body Wellness* (White River Junction, VT: Chelsea Green, 2020).
8. Anna Ciéslińska, Elzbieta Kostyra and Huub F.J. Savelkoul, 'Treating Autism Spectrum Disorder with Gluten-free and Casein-free Diet: The Underlying Microbiota-gut-brain Axis Mechanisms', *HSOA Journal of Clinical Immunology and Immunotherapy* 3 (2017): 009.
9. Matts Hanson, 'Amalgam: Hazards in Your Teeth', *Journal of Orthomolecular Psychiatry* 12, no. 3 (1983): 194–201; Patrick Störtebecker, 'Direct Transport of Mercury from the Oronasal Cavity to the Cranial Cavity as a Cause of Dental Amalgam Poisoning', *Swedish Journal of Biological Medicine* 3 (1989): 8–21; Vera D.M. Stejskal, Margit Forsbeck, Karin E. Cederbrant and Ola Asteman, 'Mercury-specific Lymphocytes: An

Indication of Mercury Allergy in Man', *Journal of Clinical Immunology* 16 (1996): 31–40.

10. Irving M. Shapiro et al., 'Neurophysiological and Neuropsychological Function in Mercury-exposed Dentists', *The Lancet* 319, no. 8282 (1982): 1147–1150; B.P. Uzzell et al., 'Chronic Low-level Mercury Exposure and Neuropsychological Functioning', *Journal of Clinical and Experimental Neuropsychology* 8, no. 5 (1982): 1147–1150.
11. 'Gold Amalgam', Geology, https://geology.com/usgs/gold.
12. Catherine Tomicic, David Vernez, Tounaba Belem and Michèle Berode, 'Human Mercury Exposure Associated with Small-scale Gold Mining in Burkina Faso', *International Archives of Occupational and Environmental Health* 84 (2011): 539–546; Justice Afrifa et al., 'The Clinical Importance of the Mercury Problem in Artisanal Small-Scale Gold Mining', *Frontiers in Public Health* 7 (2019): 131.
13. Rock and Gem, https://www.rockngem.com.
14. Dr Graeme Munro-Hall, personal communication, 15 May 2023.
15. Dr Rachel Nicoll, lecture to British Society for Ecological Medicine, London, 2015.
16. Michael Coryell et al., 'The Gut Microbiome is Required for Full Protection against Acute Arsenic Toxicity in Mouse Models', *Nature Communications* 9, no. 1 (2018): 5424.
17. Michael P. Waalkes, 'Cadmium Carcinogenesis', *Mutation Research/Fundamental and Molecular Mechanisms of Mutagenesis* 533, no. 1–2 (2003): 107–120.
18. P.D. Darbre, 'Metalloestrogens: An Emerging Class of Inorganic Xenoestrogens with Potential to Add to the Oestrogenic Burden of the Human Breast', *Journal of Applied Toxicology* 26 (2006): 191–197. https://doi.org/10.1002/jat.1135.
19. E. Blaurock-Busch et al., 'Metal Exposure in the Children of Punjab, India', *Clinical Medicine Insights: Therapeutics* 2 (2010): CMT-S5154.
20. A.M.G. Campbell, E.R. Williams and D. Barltrop, 'Motor Neurone Disease and Exposure to Lead', *Journal of Neurology, Neurosurgery & Psychiatry* 33, no. 6 (1970): 877–885.
21. Hokuto Nakata et al., 'Narrative Review of Lead Poisoning in Humans Caused by Industrial Activities and Measures Compatible with Sustainable Industrial Activities in Republic of Zambia', *Science of The Total Environment* 850 (2022): 157833.

22. R.M. Abdel-Megeed, 'Probiotics: A Promising Generation of Heavy Metal Detoxification', *Biol Trace Elem Res* 199 (2021): 2406–2413, https://doi.org/10.1007/s12011-020-02350-1.

23. P.D. Darbre, 'Aluminium and the Human Breast', *Morphologie* 100, no. 329 (2016): 65–74.

24. Daniel P. Perl, 'Relationship of Aluminum to Alzheimer's Disease', *Environmental Health Perspectives* 63 (1985): 149–153.

25. Abdel-Megeed, 'Probiotics', 2406–2413.

26. B. Vellingiri et al., 'Influence of Heavy Metals in Parkinson's Disease: An Overview', *Journal of Neurology* 269 (2022): 5798–5811.

27. Magdalena Czajka et al., 'Toxicity of Titanium Dioxide Nanoparticles in Central Nervous System', *Toxicology In Vitro* 29, no. 5 (2015): 1042–1052.

28. EFSA Panel on Food Additives and Flavourings et al., 'Scientific Opinion on the Safety Assessment of Titanium Dioxide (E171) as a Food Additive', *EFSA Journal* 19, no. 5 (2021): e06585, https://doi.org/10.2903/j.efsa.2021.6585.

Chapter Three

1. William R. MacKenzie et al., 'A Massive Outbreak in Milwaukee of Cryptosporidium Infection Transmitted through the Public Water Supply', *New England Journal of Medicine* 331, no. 3 (1994): 161–167.

2. Krishna Gopal et al., 'Chlorination Byproducts, Their Toxicodynamics and Removal from Drinking Water', *Journal of Hazardous Materials* 140, no. 1–2 (2007): 1–6, https://doi.org/10.1016/j.jhazmat.2006.10.063.

3. Susan Richardson et al., 'Occurrence, Genotoxicity and Carcinogenicity of Regulated and Emerging Disinfection By-Products in Drinking Water: A Review and Roadmap for Research', *Mutation Research/Reviews in Mutation Research* 636, no. 1–3 (2007): 178–242.

4. Kenneth P. Cantor et al., 'Drinking Water Source and Chlorination Byproducts I. Risk of Bladder Cancer', *Epidemiology* 9, no. 1 (1998): 21–28; Mariana E Hildesheim et al., 'Drinking Water Source and Chlorination Byproducts II. Risk of Colon and Rectal Cancers', *Epidemiology* 9, no. 1 (1998): 29–35; Timothy J. Doyle et al., 'The Association of Drinking Water Source and Chlorination By-Products with Cancer Incidence

Among Postmenopausal Women in Iowa: A Prospective Cohort Study', *American Journal of Public Health* 87, no. 7 (1997): 1168–1176.

5. Patrick Smeets, Gertjan J. Medema and J.C. van Dijk, 'The Dutch Secret: How to Provide Safe Drinking Water Without Chlorine in the Netherlands', *Drinking Water Engineering and Science* 2, no. 1 (2009): 1–14; Joop C. Kruithof, R. Chr. van der Leer and Wim A.M. Hijnen, 'Practical Experiences with UV Disinfection in the Netherlands', *Aqua – Journal of Water Supply: Research and Technology* 41, no. 2 (1992): 88–94.
6. Paul Connett, James Beck and H. Spedding Micklem, *The Case Against Fluoride: How Hazardous Waste Ended Up in Our Drinking Water and the Bad Science and Powerful Politics That Keep It There* (White River Junction, VT: Chelsea Green, 2012), 40.
7. L. Seppä , S. Kärkkäinen and H. Hausen. 'Caries Trends 1992–1998 in Two Low-Fluoride Finnish Towns Formerly with and without Fluoridation', *Caries Research* 34, no. 6 (2000): 462–468; W. Künzel and T. Fischer, 'Caries Prevalence after Cessation of Water Fluoridation in La Salud, Cuba', *Caries Research* 34, no. 1 (2000): 20–25.
8. John Colquhoun, 'Why I Changed My Mind About Water Fluoridation', *Perspectives in Biology and Medicine* 41, no. 1 (1997): 29–44, https://doi.org/10.1353/pbm.1997.0017; John A. Yiamouyiannis, 'Water Fluoridation and Tooth Decay: Results from the 1986–1987 National Survey of U.S. School Children', *Fluoride* 23, no.2 (1990): 55–67.
9. Connett, Beck and Micklem, *Case Against Fluoride*, 38.
10. Hardy Limeback, 'A Re-examination of the Pre-eruptive and Post-eruptive Mechanism of the Anti-caries Effects of Fluoride: Is There Any Anti-caries Benefit from Swallowing Fluoride?', *Community Dentistry and Oral Epidemiology* 27, no. 1 (1999): 62–71.
11. H.V. Churchill, 'The Occurrence of Fluorides in Some Waters of the United States', *Journal of Dental Research* 12, no. 1 (1932): 141–148, https://doi.org/10.1177/00220345320120010401.
12. Y. Lu et al., 'Effect of High-fluoride Water on Intelligence in Children', *Fluoride* 33, no. 2 (2000): 74–78.
13. Wendee Nicole, 'Denser but Not Stronger? Fluoride-Induced Bone Growth and Increased Risk of Hip Fractures', *Environmental Health Perspectives* 129, no. 7 (2007): 074001.

14. Emilie Helte et al., 'Fluoride in Drinking Water, Diet, and Urine in Relation to Bone Mineral Density and Fracture Incidence in Postmenopausal Women', *Environmental Health Perspectives* 129, no. 4 (2021): 047005.

15. Chris Neurath, 'Presentation at the 35th Conference of the International Society for Fluoride Research', 28–31 July 2022, Harbin, China. (Includes their own methodology and results, and a critique of PHE's study.)

16. Elise B. Bassin et al., 'Age-specific Fluoride Exposure in Drinking Water and Osteosarcoma (United States)', *Cancer Causes and Control* 17 (2006): 421–428.

17. Connett, Beck and Micklem, *Case Against Fluoride*, chapter 18.

18. Ann L. Choi, Guifan Sun, Ying Zhang and Philippe Grandjean, 'Developmental Fluoride Neurotoxicity: A Systematic Review and Meta-analysis', *Environmental Health Perspectives* 120, no. 10 (2012): 1362–1368; Anna L. Choi et al., 'Association of Lifetime Exposure to Fluoride and Cognitive Functions in Chinese Children: A Pilot Study', *Neurotoxicology and Teratology* 47 (2015): 96–101; Philippe Grandjean, 'Developmental Fluoride Neurotoxicity: An Updated Review', *Environmental Health* 18, no. 1 (2019): 1–17.

19. Christine Till et al., 'Community Water Fluoridation and Urinary Fluoride Concentrations in a National Sample of Pregnant Women in Canada', *Environmental Health Perspectives* 126, no. 10 (2018): 107001; Abduweli Uyghurturk et al., 'Maternal and Fetal Exposures to Fluoride during Mid-gestation Among Pregnant Women in Northern California', *Environmental Health* 19, no. 1 (2020): 1–9.

20. Christine Till et al., 'Fluoride Exposure from Infant Formula and Child IQ in a Canadian Birth Cohort', *Environment International* 134 (2020): 105315.

21. Morteza Bashash et al., 'Prenatal Fluoride Exposure and Cognitive Outcomes in Children at 4 and 6–12 years of Age in Mexico', *Environmental Health Perspectives* 125, no. 9 (2017): 097017.

22. Alejandra Cantoral et al., 'Dietary Fluoride Intake During Pregnancy and Neurodevelopment in Toddlers: A Prospective Study in the Progress Cohort', *Neurotoxicology* 87 (2021): 86–93.

23. Cantoral et al., 'Dietary Fluoride Intake During Pregnancy', 86–93.

24. Rivka Green et al., 'Association Between Maternal Fluoride Exposure During Pregnancy and IQ Scores in Offspring in Canada', *JAMA*

Pediatrics 173, no. 10 (2019): 940–948; Q. Xiang et al., 'Effect of Fluoride in Drinking Water on Children's Intelligence', *Fluoride* 36, no. 2 (2003): 84–94; Philippe Grandjean et al., 'A Benchmark Dose Analysis for Maternal Pregnancy Urine-Fluoride and IQ in Children', *Risk Analysis* 42, no. 3 (2022): 439–449.

25. L. Valdez Jiménez et al., 'In Utero Exposure to Fluoride and Cognitive Development Delay in Infants', *Neurotoxicology* 59 (2017): 65–70.

26. Morteza Bashash et al., 'Prenatal Fluoride Exposure and Attention Deficit Hyperactivity Disorder (ADHD) Symptoms in Children at 6–12 Years of Age in Mexico City', *Environment International* 121 (2018): 658–666.

27. Connett, Beck and Micklem, *Case Against Fluoride*, chapter 19.

28. Meaghan Hall et al., 'Fluoride Exposure and Hypothyroidism in a Canadian Pregnancy Cohort', *Science of The Total Environment* 869 (2023): 161149.

29. Carly V. Goodman et al., 'Iodine Status Modifies the Association Between Fluoride Exposure in Pregnancy and Preschool Boys' Intelligence', *Nutrients* 14, no. 14 (2022): 2920.

30. Jennifer Luke, 'Fluoride Deposition in the Aged Human Pineal Gland', *Caries Research* 35, no. 2 (2001): 125–128; Jennifer Anne Luke, 'The Effect of Fluoride on the Physiology of the Pineal Gland' (PhD diss., University of Surrey, 1997).

31. Connett, Beck and Micklem, *Case Against Fluoride*, 166.

32. Elizabeth A. McDonagh, 'Rapid Response: Fluoride – a Harmful Mineral Element', *British Medical Journal* 335 (2007): 699, https://doi.org/10.1136/bmj.39318.562951.BE.

33. McDonagh, 'Rapid Response', 699.

34. Joel Bakan, *The Corporation: The Pathological Pursuit of Profit and Power* (London: Hachette, 2012).

35. Christopher Bryson, *The Fluoride Deception* (New York: Seven Stories Press, 2004).

36. Connett, Beck and Micklem, *Case Against Fluoride*, 264–5.

37. Will McCallum, *How to Give up Plastic* (New York: Penguin Random House, 2019).

38. Natalie Fée, *How to Save the World for Free* (London: Laurence King, 2021), 11, 16, 48–49, 66–69, 89.

39. My thanks to Tyler Luke Cunningham for drawing my attention to this documentary.
40. Julia R. Varshavsky et al., 'Dietary Sources of Cumulative Phthalates Exposure Among the US General Population in NHANES 2005–2014', *Environment International* 115 (2018): 417–429.
41. Dr Pol de Saedeleer, 'Presentation to British Society for Ecological Medicine', 23 June 2023, London, UK; Sailas Benjamin et al., 'Phthalates Impact Human Health: Epidemiological Evidences and Plausible Mechanism of Action', *Journal of Hazardous Materials* 340 (2017): 360–383; Waleed Adawi, Nishadh Sutaria and Varsha Parthasarathy, '35256 Urinary Mono-benzyl-phthalate Levels are Associated with Increasing Psoriasis Severity in US Adults', *Journal of the American Academy of Dermatology* 87, no. 3 (2022): AB125; Henrieta Hlisníková et al., 'Effects and Mechanisms of Phthalates' Action on Reproductive Processes and Reproductive Health: A Literature Review', *International Journal of Environmental Research and Public Health* 17, no. 18 (2020): 6811.
42. Haitao Zhu et al., 'Growth-promoting Effect of Bisphenol A on Neuroblastoma In Vitro And In Vivo', *Journal of Pediatric Surgery* 44, no. 4 (2009): 672–680.
43. Maurício Martins da Silva et al., 'Inhibition of Type 1 Iodothyronine Deiodinase by Bisphenol A', *Hormone and Metabolic Research* 51, no. 10 (2019): 671–677.
44. Ming-Yu Xie, 'Exposure to Bisphenol A and the Development of Asthma: A Systematic Review of Cohort Studies', *Reproductive Toxicology* 65 (2016): 224–229.
45. David Melzer et al., 'Association of Urinary Bisphenol A Concentration with Heart Disease: Evidence from NHANES 2003/06', *PloS One* 5, no. 1 (2010): e8673.
46. Datis Kharrazian, 'The Potential Roles of Bisphenol A (BPA) Pathogenesis in Autoimmunity', *Autoimmune Diseases* 2014 (2014).
47. Pol de Saedeleer, 'Presentation to British Society for Ecological Medicine'.
48. Pol de Saedeleer.
49. Jennifer C. Hartle, Ana Navas-Acien and Robert S. Lawrence, 'The Consumption of Canned Food and Beverages and Urinary Bisphenol A Concentrations in NHANES 2003–2008', *Environmental Research* 150 (2016): 375–382.

50. McCallum, *How to Give up Plastic*, 86.
51. Toxic-Free Future, 'Toxic Convenience: The hidden Costs of Forever Chemicals in Stain- and Water-Resistant Products', 26 January 2022.
52. Alden Wicker, *To Dye For* (New York: Putnam, 2023).
53. Amelia Twine, personal communication, 12 September 2023.
54. Russ Carrington, personal communication, 20 July 2023.
55. Rebecca Hosking, personal communication, July 2023.
56. My thanks to Amelia Twine, op cit, for much of the information contained in this paragraph.
57. Rebecca Burgess, *Fibershed* (White River Junction, VT: Chelsea Green, 2019).
58. My thanks to Emma Hague of South West England Fibreshed for checking this section.
59. Fée, *How to Save the World for Free*, 143.
60. Jacqui and Michael: thanks for the inspiration!
61. Alden Wicker, *To Dye For*, 87.
62. Chunyuan Fei et al., 'Perfluorinated Chemicals and Fetal Growth: A Study Within the Danish National Birth Cohort', *Environmental Health Perspectives* 115, no. 11 (2007): 1677–1682.
63. Chunjie Xia et al., 'Per- and Polyfluoroalkyl Substances in North American School Uniforms', *Environmental Science & Technology* 56, no. 19 (2022): 13845–13857.
64. Kathryn M. Rodgers et al., 'How Well Do Product Labels Indicate the Presence of PFAS in Consumer Items Used by Children and Adolescents?', *Environmental Science & Technology* 56, no. 10 (2022): 6294–6304.
65. Fire Brigades Union, 'Fire Contaminants Linked to Significant Physical and Mental Health Issues Among UK Firefighters', 10 January 2023, https://www.fbu.org.uk/news/2023/01/10/fire-contaminants-linked-significant-physical-and-mental-health-issues-among-uk.
66. Min Joo Kim et al., 'Association Between Perfluoroalkyl Substances Exposure and Thyroid Function in Adults: A Meta-analysis', *PloS One* 13, no. 5 (2018): e0197244.
67. Cathrine Carlsen Bach et al., 'Perfluoroalkyl and Polyfluoroalkyl Substances and Human Fetal Growth: A Systematic Review', *Critical Reviews in Toxicology* 45, no. 1 (2015): 53–67.

68. Sarah S. Knox et al., 'Implications of Early Menopause in Women Exposed to Perfluorocarbons', *The Journal of Clinical Endocrinology & Metabolism* 96, no. 6 (2011): 1747–1753.

69. Xia et al., 'Per- and Polyfluoroalkyl Substances', 13845–13857.

70. Sung Kyun Park et al., 'Per- and Polyfluoroalkyl Substances and Incident Diabetes in Midlife Women: The Study of Women's Health Across the Nation (SWAN)', *Diabetologia* 65, no. 7 (2022): 1157–1168.

71. Jesse A. Goodrich et al., 'Exposure to Perfluoroalkyl Substances and Risk of Hepatocellular Carcinoma in a Multiethnic Cohort', *JHEP Reports* 4, no. 10 (2022): 100550.

72. Vladislav Obsekov, Linda G. Kahn and Leonardo Trasande, 'Leveraging Systematic Reviews to Explore Disease Burden and Costs of Per- and Polyfluoroalkyl Substance Exposures in the United States', *Exposure and Health* 15, no. 2 (2023): 373–394.

73. Viet Tung Nguyen, Martin Reinhard and Gin Yew-Hoong Karina, 'Occurrence and Source Characterization of Perfluorochemicals in an Urban Watershed,' *Chemosphere* 82, no. 9 (2011): 1277–1285.

74. John Naish, 'The Toxic "Forever Chemicals" That Could Be Lurking In Your Home', *The Times*, 28 September 2022.

75. Naish, 'The Toxic "Forever Chemicals"'.

76. Bakan, *The Corporation*.

77. Wicker, *To Dye For*, 85.

78. Esme Stallard and Jonah Fisher, 'Raw Sewage Spills into England Rivers and Seas Doubles in 2023', BBC News, 27 March 2024, https://www.bbc.co.uk/news/science-environment-68665335.

79. Gill Plimmer and Ella Hollowood, 'Water Companies Pay £2.5bn in Dividends in Two Years as Debt Climbs by £8.2bn', *Financial Times*, 15 April 2024, https://www.ft.com/content/c3cdfefb-c912-4699-bb7f-72c5c6515757.

80. Guy Singh-Watson, 'Water, Unbridled Capitalism and Geese', *Wicked Leeks*, 22 June 2023, https://wickedleeks.riverford.co.uk/opinion/water-unbridled-capitalism-and-geese.

81. John L. Wilkinson et al., 'Pharmaceutical Pollution of the World's Rivers', *Proceedings of the National Academy of Sciences* 119, no. 8 (2022): e2113947119.

82. Thomas H. Miller et al., 'A Review of the Pharmaceutical Exposome in Aquatic Fauna', *Environmental Pollution* 239 (2018): 129–146.

83. Wilkinson et al., 'Pharmaceutical Pollution', e2113947119.

84. A. Elaine McKeown and George Bugyi, *Impact of Water Pollution on Human Health and Environmental Sustainability* (Hershey, PA: Information Science Reference, 2016), 61.

Chapter Four

1. Stephen T. Holgate, '"Every Breath We Take: The Lifelong Impact of Air Pollution"– A Call for Action', *Clinical Medicine* 17, no. 1 (2017): 8; Zeinab Al-Rekabi et al., 'Uncovering the Cytotoxic Effects of Air Pollution with Multi-modal Imaging of In Vitro Respiratory Models', *Royal Society Open Science* 10, no. 4 (2023): 221426; Clean Air Fund, https://www.cleanairfund.org.

2. European Environment Agency, 'Health Impacts of Air Pollution in Europe, 2022', EEA, last modified 20 November 2023, https://www.eea.europa.eu/publications/air-quality-in-europe-2022/health-impacts-of-air-pollution.

3. Christine Ro, 'Could "Flight Shame" Lead to Green Holiday Travel? Meet the Companies Prompting Employees to Choose Trains over Planes', BBC, 18 September 2019, https://www.bbc.com/worklife/article/20190918-some-firms-give-more-time-off-to-those-who-shun-plane-travel.

4. Ro, 'Could "Flight Shame" Lead to Green Holiday Travel?'

5. Katja M Bendtsen, Elizabeth Bengtsen, Anne T. Saber and Ulla Vogel, 'A Review of Health Effects Associated with Exposure to Jet Engine Emissions In and Around Airports', *Environmental Health* 20, no. 1 (2021): 1–21.

6. Jeremy Thompson and Honor Anthony, 'The Health Effects of Waste Incinerators', *British Society for Ecological Medicine*, 2005.

7. Damian Carrington, 'Microplastic Raining Down on Cities, Say Scientists Amid Call for Urgent Research', *Guardian*, 28 December 2019, 5.

8. Carrington, 'Microplastic Raining Down on Cities', 5.

9. Christoph Steffen et al., 'Acute Childhood Leukaemia and Environmental Exposure to Potential Sources of Benzene and Other Hydrocarbons; A Case-control Study', *Occupational and Environmental Medicine* 61, no.

9 (2004): 773–778; Pauline Brosselin et al., 'Acute Childhood Leukaemia and Residence Next to Petrol Stations and Automotive Repair Garages: the ESCALE study (SFCE)', *Occupational and Environmental Medicine* 66, no. 9 (2009): 598–606.

10. International Agency for Research on Cancer.

11. Peter Kaatsch, 'Epidemiology of Childhood Cancer', *Cancer Treatment Reviews* 36, no. 4 (2010): 277–285.

12. Theodore I. Lidsky and Jay S. Schneider, 'Lead Neurotoxicity in Children: Basic Mechanisms and Clinical Correlates', *Brain* 126, no. 1 (2003): 5–19.

13. Zhang, Zili, Jian Wang and Wenju Lu, 'Exposure to Nitrogen Dioxide and Chronic Obstructive Pulmonary Disease (COPD) in Adults: A Systematic Review and Meta-analysis', *Environmental Science and Pollution Research* 25 (2018): 15133–15145.

14. Sara M. May and James T.C. Li, 'Burden of Chronic Obstructive Pulmonary Disease: Healthcare Costs and Beyond', *Allergy and Asthma Proceedings* 36, no. 1 (2015): 4.

15. Tim Smedley, *Clearing the Air: The Beginning and the End of Air Pollution* (London: Bloomsbury, 2019), 17–18.

16. Smedley, *Clearing the Air*, 76–77.

17. Ning Li et al., 'A Work Group Report on Ultrafine Particles (American Academy of Allergy, Asthma & Immunology): Why Ambient Ultrafine and Engineered Nanoparticles Should Receive Special Attention For Possible Adverse Health Outcomes in Human Subjects', *Journal of Allergy and Clinical Immunology* 138, no. 2 (2016): 386–396.

18. C. Arden Pope III et al., 'Lung Cancer, Cardiopulmonary Mortality, and Long-Term Exposure to Fine Particulate Air Pollution', *JAMA* 287, no. 9 (2002): 1132–1141.

19. Richard B. Hayes et al., 'PM2. 5 Air Pollution and Cause-Specific Cardiovascular Disease Mortality', *International Journal of Epidemiology* 49, no. 1 (2020): 25–35.

20. Lilian Calderón-Garcidueñas et al., 'Air Pollution, Combustion and Friction Derived Nanoparticles, and Alzheimer's Disease in Urban Children and Young Adults', *Journal of Alzheimer's Disease* 70, no. 2 (2019): 343–360.

21. Norrice M. Liu et al., 'Evidence for the Presence of Air Pollution Nanoparticles in Placental Tissue Cells', *Science of The Total Environment* 751 (2021): 142235.

22. Holgate, '"Every Breath We Take"', 8.

23. Rossa Brugha and Jonathan Grigg, 'Urban Air Pollution and Respiratory Infections', *Paediatric Respiratory Reviews* 15, no. 2 (2014): 194–199.

24. Jonathan Grigg, 'Helping London's Children Breathe More Easily: How Queen Mary Research Influenced the Introduction of the Ultra Low Emission Zone', Blizard Institute, Queen Mary University, London, 16 May 2021.

25. Sadiq Khan, *Breathe: Tackling the Climate Emergency* (London: Hutchinson Heinemann, 2023) 56.

26. Unicef UK, 'The Toxic School Run', Unicef UK Research Briefing (2019).

27. Nathan R. Gray, Alastair C. Lewis and Sarah J. Moller, 'Deprivation Based Inequality in NO x Emissions in England', *Environmental Science: Advances* 2, no. 9 (2023): 1261–1272.

28. Li Wang et al., 'Air Quality Strategies on Public Health and Health Equity in Europe – a Systematic Review', *International Journal of Environmental Research and Public Health* 13, no. 12 (2016): 1196.

29. A. Karamanos et al., 'Associations Between Air Pollutants and Blood Pressure in an Ethnically Diverse Cohort of Adolescents in London, England', *Plos One* 18, no. 2 (2023): e0279719.

30. Bert Brunekreef and Stephen T. Holgate, 'Air pollution and Health', *The Lancet* 360, no. 9341 (2002): 1233–1242.

31. Dick van Steenis, 'Airborne Pollutants and Acute Health Effects', *The Lancet* 345, no. 8954 (1995): 923.

32. House of Commons, Environment, Food and Rural Affairs, written evidence, 11 May 2006.

33. Kelly Ng, 'Thailand: 10 million Sought Treatment for Pollution-Related Illnesses in 2023', BBC News, 6 March 2024, https://www.bbc.co.uk/news/world-asia-68487230.

34. Gary Fuller, Stav Friedman and Ian Mudway, *Impacts of Air Pollution Across the Life Course – Evidence Highlight Note*, (London: Imperial College London, Environmental Research Group, 2023); Dean E. Schraufnagel et al., 'Air Pollution and Noncommunicable Diseases:

A Review by the Forum of International Respiratory Societies' Environmental Committee, Part 2: Air Pollution and Organ Systems', *Chest* 155, no. 2 (2019): 417-426; Karn Vohra et al., 'Global Mortality from Outdoor Fine Particle Pollution Generated by Fossil Fuel Combustion: Results from GEOS-Chem', *Environmental Research* 195 (2021): 110754.

35. Teumzghi F. Mebrahtu et al., 'The Effects of Exposure to NO_2, PM2. 5 and PM10 on Health Service Attendances with Respiratory Illnesses: A Time-series Analysis', Environmental Pollution 333 (2023): 122123.

36. Fuller, Friedman and Mudway, 'Impacts of Air Pollution', 2.

37. Survival International, personal communication, 20 June 2023.

38. Tim Smedley, *Clearing the Air*, 197–205.

39. Ian S. Mudway et al., 'Impact of London's Low Emission Zone on Air Quality and Children's Respiratory Health: A Sequential Annual Cross-sectional Study', *The Lancet Public Health* 4, no. 1 (2019): e28–e40; Rosemary C. Chamberlain et al., 'Health Effects of Low Emission and Congestion Charging Zones: A Systematic Review', *The Lancet Public Health* 8, no. 7 (2023): e559–e574.

40. Alexander Massey, personal communication, 28 September 2023.

41. Rob Verkerk, Alliance for Natural Health, personal communication, 27 October 2023.

Chapter Five

1. Martin J. Gardner et al., 'Results of Case-control Study of Leukaemia and Lymphoma Among Young People Near Sellafield Nuclear Plant in West Cumbria', *British Medical Journal* 300, no. 6722 (1990): 423–429; Martin J. Gardner et al., 'Follow Up Study of Children Born to Mothers Resident in Seascale, West Cumbria (birth cohort)', *British Medical Journal (Clinical Research Edition)* 295, no. 6602 (1987): 822–827; J.W. Stather et al., 'The Risk of Leukemia in Seascale from Radiation Exposure', *Health Physics* 55, no. 2 (1988): 471–481.

2. Christopher Busby, 'Is There Evidence of Adverse Health Effects Near US Nuclear Installations? Infant Mortality in Coastal Communities near The Diablo Canyon Nuclear Power Station in California, 1989–2012', *Jacobs Journal of Epidemiology and Preventive Medicine* 2, no.3 (2016): 030; Peter J. Baker and D.G. Hoel, 'Meta-analysis of Standardized Incidence and Mortality Rates of Childhood Leukaemia in Proximity to Nuclear Facilities', *European Journal of Cancer Care* 16, no. 4 (2007): 355–363.

3. Chris Busby, *Wings of Death: Nuclear Pollution and Human Health* (Aberystwyth: Green Audit Books, 1995), 58.
4. Alice Stewart, Josefine Webb and David Hewitt, 'A Survey of Childhood Malignancies', *British Medical Journal* 1, no. 5086 (1958): 1495.
5. Brian MacMahon 'Prenatal X-ray Exposure and Childhood Cancer', *Journal of the National Cancer Institute* 28, no. 5 (1962): 1173–1191.
6. Jay M. Gould and Benjamin A. Goldman, *Deadly Deceit: Low Level Radiation, High Level Cover-up* (New York: Four Walls Eight Windows, 1991), 15–17.
7. Gould and Goldman, *Deadly Deceit*, 15.
8. Gould and Goldman , 39.
9. Keith Schneider, 'Severe Accidents at Nuclear Plant Were Kept Secret up to 31 Years', *New York Times*, 1 October 1988.
10. Gould and Goldman, *Deadly Deceit*, 48–51.
11. Gould and Goldman, 175–7.
12. Gould and Goldman, 50–51.
13. Busby, *Wings of Death*, 236–272.
14. Chris Busby and Mireille de Messieres, 'Cancer Near Trawsfynydd Nuclear Power Station in Wales, UK: A Cross Sectional Cohort Study', *Environmental Research SIA*, 6 March 2015.
15. P.M. Sheehan and Irene B. Hillary, 'An Unusual Cluster of Babies with Down's Syndrome Born to Former Pupils of an Irish Boarding School', *British Medical Journal (Clinical research ed.)* 287, no. 6403 (1983): 1428.
16. Richard Bramhall, Low Level Radiation Campaign, personal communication, 10 November 23.
17. Chris Busby and Molly Scott Cato, 'Increases in Leukemia in Infants in Wales and Scotland Following Chernobyl: Evidence for Errors in Statutory Risk Estimates', *Energy & Environment* 11, no. 2 (2000): 127–139.
18. Busby, *Wings of Death*, 89.
19. Busby, 89.
20. Derek Jakeman, 'New Estimates of Radioactive Discharges from Sellafield', *British Medical Journal* 293, no. 6549 (20 September 1986): 760.
21. Abram Petkau, 'Radiation Carcinogenesis From A Membrane Perspective', *Acta Physiologica Scandinavica. Supplementum* 492 (1980): 81–90.

22. Joseph J. Mangano and Janette D. Sherman, 'Elevated In Vivo Strontium-90 from Nuclear Weapons Test Fallout Among Cancer Decedents: A Case-control Study of Deciduous Teeth', *International Journal of Health Services* 41, no. 1 (2011): 137–158.

23. N.A. Gillett et al., 'Strontium-90 Induced Bone Tumours in Beagle Dogs: Effects of Route of Exposure and Dose Rate', *International Journal of Radiation Biology* 61, no. 6 (1992): 821–831; C.S. Klusek, 'Strontium-90 in Food and Bone from Fallout', *Journal of Environmental Quality* 16, no. 3 (1987): 195–199; Harmen Bijwaard, Marco J.P. Brugmans and Henk P. Leenhouts, 'Two-mutation Models For Bone Cancer Due to Radium, Strontium And Plutonium', *Radiation Research* 162, no. 2 (2004): 171–184.

24. Yasushi Nishiwaki et al., 'Effects of Radioactive Fallout on the Pregnant Woman and the Fetus', *International Journal of Environmental Studies* 2, no. 1–4 (1971): 277–289; Busby, *Wings of Death*, 219.

25. Alexandra Dawe at al., *Nuclear Scars: The Lasting Legacies of Chernobyl and Fukushima* (Amsterdam: Greenpeace International, 2016).

26. V.A. Stsjazhko et al., 'Childhood Thyroid Cancer Since Accident At Chernobyl', *British Medical Journal* 310, no. 6982 (1995): 801.

27. Toshihide Tsuda, Akiko Tokinobu, Eiji Yamamoto and Etsuji Suzuki, 'Thyroid Cancer Detection By Ultrasound Among Residents Ages 18 Years and Younger In Fukushima, Japan: 2011 to 2014', *Epidemiology* 27, no. 3 (2016): 316.

28. Inge Schmitz-Feuerhake, Christopher Busby and Sebastian Pflugbeil, 'Genetic Radiation Risks: A Neglected Topic in the Low Dose Debate', *Environmental Health and Toxicology* 31 (2016).

29. Busby, *Wings of Death*, 234.

30. Chris Busby and M.E. de Messieres, 'Miscarriages and Congenital Conditions in Offspring of Veterans of the British Nuclear Atmospheric Test Programme', *Epidemiology (sunnyvale)* 4 (2014): 172.

31. Chris Busby and Aleksandra Fucic, 'Ionizing Radiation and Children's Health: Conclusions', *Acta Paediatrica* 95 (2006): 81–85.

32. Richard Bramhall, Low Level Radiation Campaign, personal communication, 10 November 2023.

33. Chris Busby, 'Uranium Epidemiology', *Jacobs Journal of Epidemiology and Preventive Medicine* 1, no.2 (2015): 009; Gould and Goldman, *Deadly Deceit*, 21.

34. Chris Busby, 'Uranium Weapons Being Employed in Ukraine Have Significantly Increased Uranium Levels in the Air in the UK ', *Environmental Research SIA*, 14 March 2023, https://doi.org/10.21203/rs.3.rs-2681787/v1.
35. Busby, 'Uranium Epidemiology', 009.
36. Bramhall, personal communication.
37. Busby, 'Uranium Epidemiology', 009.
38. Bramhall, personal communication.
39. Stewart, Webb and Hewitt, 'A Survey of Childhood Malignancies', 1495.
40. Busby, *Wings of Death*, 123.
41. Shoji Sawada, 'Cover-up of the Effects of Internal Exposure By Residual Radiation from the atomic Bombing of Hiroshima and Nagasaki', *Medicine, Conflict and Survival* 23, no. 1 (2007): 58–74.
42. Chris Busby, 'The Hiroshima A-Bomb Black Rain and the Lifespan Study; A Resolution of the Enigma', *Cancer Investigation* 39, no. 10 (2021): 902–907.
43. Chris Busby, 'Child Health and Ionizing Radiation: Science, Politics and European Law', *Pediatric Dimensions* 2 (2017): 1–4.
44. Richard Bramhall, 'The Chernobyl Deniers Use Far Too Simple A Measure of Radiation Risk', *Guardian*, 20 April 2011.
45. Chris Busby, 'Ionizing Radiation and Cancer: The Failure of the Risk Model', *Cancer Treatment and Research Communications* 31 (2022): 100565.
46. Busby, *Wings of Death*, 184–5.
47. Gould and Goldman, *Deadly Deceit*, 96.
48. Chris Busby, 'Very Low Dose Fetal Exposure to Chernobyl Contamination Resulted in Increases in Infant Leukemia in Europe and Raises Questions About Current Radiation Risk Models', *International Journal of Environmental Research and Public Health* 6, no. 12 (2009): 3105–3114.
49. Chris Busby, Mireille de Messieres and Saoirse Morgan, 'Infant and Perinatal Mortality and Stillbirths near Hinkley Point Nuclear Power Station in Somerset, 2005–1993; an Epidemiological Investigation of Causation', *Jacobs Journal of Epidemiology and Preventive Medicine* (2015).

Chapter Six

1. Jessica A. Adams et al., 'Effect of Mobile Telephones on Sperm Quality: A Systematic Review and Meta-analysis', *Environment International* 70 (2014): 106–112.

2. Rebecca L. Siegel et al., 'Global Patterns and Trends in Colorectal Cancer Incidence in Young Adults', *Gut* (2019): gutjnl-2019; J. Gandhi et al., 'Population-based Study Demonstrating an Increase in Colorectal Cancer in Young Patients', *Journal of British Surgery* 104, no. 8 (2017): 1063–1068.

3. Magda Havas, 'Analysis of Health and Environmental Effects of Proposed San Francisco Earthlink Wi-fi Network', *Commissioned by SNAFU (San Francisco Neighborhood Antenna Free Union) and presented to Board of Supervisors, City and Country of San Francisco* (2007).

4. M. Bevington, *Electromagnetic Sensitivity and Electromagnetic Hypersensitivity: A Summary* (Milton Keynes: Capability Books, 2013), 7.

5. Martin L. Pall, 'Wi-Fi is an Important Threat to Human Health', *Environmental Research* 164 (2018): 405–416.

6. Environmental Health Trust, 'Airpods Health and Safety FAQS', 8 March 2020, https://ehtrust.org/airpods-facts-health-effects-of-wireless-radiation-to-the-brain.

7. Krzysztof Gryz, Jolanta Karpowicz and Patryk Zradziński, 'Evaluation of the Influence of Magnetic Field on Female Users of an Induction Hob in Ergonomically Sound Exposure Situations', *Bioelectromagnetics* 41, no. 7 (2020): 500–510.

8. Carlo Valerio Bellieni et al., 'Electromagnetic Fields in Neonatal Incubators: The Reasons For An Alert', *The Journal of Maternal-Fetal & Neonatal Medicine* 32, no. 4 (2019): 695–699.

9. Gerd Oberfeld, 'Environmental Epidemiological Study of Cancer Incidence in the Municipalities of Hausmannstätten & Vasoldsberg (Austria)', (2008).

10. B. Blake Levitt and Henry Lai, 'Biological Effects from Exposure to Electromagnetic Radiation Emitted By Cell Tower Base Stations and Other Antenna Arrays', *Environmental Reviews* 18, (2010): 369–395.

11. International Commission on Non-Ionizing Radiation Protection, 'Guidelines for Limiting Exposure to Electromagnetic Fields (100 kHz to 300 GHz)', *Health Physics* 118, no. 5 (2020): 483–524.

12. Nancy Wertheimer and E.D. Leeper, 'Electrical Wiring Configurations and Childhood Cancer', *American Journal of Epidemiology* 109, no. 3

(1979): 273–284; Gerald Draper et al., 'Childhood Cancer in Relation to Distance from High Voltage Power Lines in England and Wales: A Case-control Study', *British Medical Journal* 330, no. 7503 (2005): 1290.

13. Chris Busby, 'Childhood Leukemia, Atmospheric Test Fallout and high Voltage Power Distribution Lines', *Pediatric Dimensions* (2017): 1943–77; A. P. Fews et al., 'Increased Exposure to Pollutant Aerosols Under High Voltage Power Lines', *International Journal of Radiation Biology* 75, no. 12 (1999).
14. Zothansiama et al., 'Impact of Radiofrequency Radiation On DNA Damage and Antioxidants in Peripheral Blood Lymphocytes of Humans Residing in the Vicinity of Mobile Phone Base Stations', *Electromagnetic Biology and Medicine* 36, no. 3 (2017): 295–305.
15. Jerry L. Phillips, Narendra Pal Singh and H. Lai, 'Electromagnetic Fields and DNA Damage', *Pathophysiology* 16, no. 2–3 (2009): 79–88.
16. M. Blank, *Overpowered: What Science Tells Us About the Dangers of Cell Phones and other Wifi-age Devices* (New York: Seven Stories Press, 2014), 54–55.
17. Claudia Schwarz et al., 'Radiofrequency Electromagnetic Fields (UMTS, 1,950 MHz) Induce Genotoxic Effects In Vitro in Human Fibroblasts but Not in Lymphocytes', *International Archives of Occupational and Environmental Health* 81 (2008): 755–767.
18. Dimitris J. Panagopoulos et al., 'Humanmade Electromagnetic Fields: Ion Forcedoscillation and Voltagegated Ion Channel Dysfunction, Oxidative Stress and DNA Damage', *International Journal of Oncology* 59, no. 5 (2021): 1–16.
19. Martin L. Pall, 'Microwave Electromagnetic Fields Act By Activating Voltage-gated Calcium Channels: Why the Current International Safety Standards Do Not Predict Biological Hazard', *Recent Res Devel Mol Cell Biol* 7 (2014): 1–15.
20. G. Hajnóczky et al., 'Mitochondrial Calcium Signalling and Cell Death: Approaches for Assessing the Role of Mitochondrial Ca2+ Uptake In Apoptosis', *Cell Calcium* 40, no. 5–6 (2006): 553–560.
21. Blank, *Overpowered*, 241.
22. D. Davis, *Disconnect: The Truth About Cellphone Radiation, What the Industry is Doing to Hide it and How to Protect Your Family* (New York: Plume Books, 2011), 21.
23. Olle Johansson and Einar Flydal, 'Health Risk from Wireless? The Debate is Over', *ElectromagneticHealth*, https://electromagnetichealth.

org/electromagnetic-health-blog/article-by-professor-olle-johansson-health-risk-from-wireless-the-debate-is-over.

24. Daniel T. DeBaun and Ryan P. DeBaun, *Radiation Nation: Fallout of Modern Technology* (Princeton, NJ: Icaro Publishing, 2017), 114–5.

25. Lennart Hardell et al., 'Case-control Study of the Association Between Malignant Brain Tumours Diagnosed Between 2007 and 2009 and Mobile and Cordless Phone Use', *International Journal of Oncology* 43, no. 6 (2013): 1833–1845.

26. Naomi Oreskes and Erik M. Conway, *Merchants of Doubt: How a Handful of Scientists Obscured The Truth on Issues from Tobacco Smoke to Global Warming* (New York: Bloomsbury, 2010), 136 et seq.

27. Sandro La Vignera et al., 'Effects of the Exposure to Mobile Phones on Male Reproduction: A Review of the Literature', *Journal of Andrology* 33, no. 3 (2012): 350–356.

28. Mehmet Esref Alkis et al., 'Single-strand DNA Breaks and Oxidative Changes in Rat Testes Exposed to Radiofrequency Radiation Emitted from Cellular Phones', *Biotechnology & Biotechnological Equipment* 33, no. 1 (2019): 1733–1740.

29. De-Kun Li et al., 'A Population-based Prospective Cohort Study of Personal Exposure to Magnetic Fields During Pregnancy and the Risk of Miscarriage', *Epidemiology* (2002): 9–20.

30. Leif G. Salford et al., 'Nerve Cell Damage in Mammalian Brain After Exposure to Microwaves from GSM Mobile Phones', *Environmental Health Perspectives* 111, no. 7 (2003): 881–883.

31. Da-peng Jiang et al., 'Electromagnetic Pulse Exposure Induces Overexpression of Beta Amyloid Protein in Rats', *Archives of Medical Research* 44, no. 3 (2013): 178–184.

32. Anke Huss, Adrian Spoerri, Matthias Egger and Martin Röösli for the Swiss National Cohort Study, 'Residence Near Power Lines and Mortality from Neurodegenerative Diseases: Longitudinal Study of the Swiss Population', *American Journal of Epidemiology* 169, no. 2 (2009): 167–175.

33. Allan H. Frey, Sondra R. Feld and Barbara Frey, 'Neural Function and Behavior: Defining the Relationship', *Annals of the New York Academy of Sciences* 247, no. 433 (1975); Allan H. Frey, 'Headaches from Cellular Telephones: Are They Real and What Are the Implications?', *Environmental Health Perspectives* 106, no. 3 (1998): 101–103; Henrietta Nittby et al., 'Radiofrequency and Extremely Low-Frequency Electromagnetic

Field Effects on the Blood-brain Barrier', *Electromagnetic Biology and Medicine* 27, no. 2 (2008): 103–126.

34. Dariusz Leszczynski et al., 'Non-thermal Activation of the hsp27/p38MAPK Stress Pathway by Mobile Phone Radiation in Human Endothelial Cells: Molecular Mechanism for Cancer-and Blood-brain Barrier related Effects', *Differentiation* 70, no. 2–3 (2002): 120–129.
35. Sarah Al-Bachari et al., 'Blood–brain Barrier Leakage is Increased in Parkinson's Disease', *Frontiers in Physiology* 11 (2020): 593026.
36. Davis, *Disconnect*, 160–164.
37. Samuel Milham, 'Amyotrophic Lateral Sclerosis (Lou Gehrig's Disease) Is Caused by Electric Currents Applied to or Induced in the Body: It Is an Iatrogenic Disease of Athletes Caused by Use of Electrotherapy Devices', *Medical Hypotheses* 74, no. 6 (2010), 1086–1087, https://doi.org/10.1016/j.mehy.2010.01.033.
38. Martin L. Pall, 'Microwave Frequency Electromagnetic Fields (EMFs) Produce Widespread Neuropsychiatric Effects Including Depression', *Journal of Chemical Neuroanatomy* 75 (2016): 43–51.
39. A.A. Kolodynski and V.V. Kolodynska, 'Motor and Psychological Functions of School Children Living in the Area of the Skrunda Radio Location Station in Latvia', *Science of the Total Environment* 180, no. 1 (1996): 87–93; Sultan Ayoub Meo et al., 'Mobile Phone Base Station Tower Settings Adjacent to School Buildings: Impact on Students' Cognitive Health', *American Journal of Men's Health* 13, no. 1 (2019): 1557988318816914.
40. Jean M. Twenge et al., 'Increases in Depressive Symptoms, Suicide-related Outcomes, and Suicide Rates Among US Adolescents After 2010 and Links to Increased New Media Screen Time', *Clinical Psychological Science* 6, no. 1 (2018): 3–17; Stephen F. Perry et al., 'Environmental Power-frequency Magnetic Fields and Suicide', *Health Physics* 41, no. 2 (1981): 267–277.
41. L. Lloyd Morgan, Santosh Kesari, and Devra Lee Davis, 'Why Children Absorb More Microwave Radiation Than Adults: The Consequences', *Journal of Microscopy and Ultrastructure* 2, no. 4 (2014): 197–204.
42. David A. Savitz et al., 'Case-control Study of Childhood Cancer and Exposure to 60-Hz Magnetic Fields', *American Journal of Epidemiology* 128, no. 1 (1988): 21–38.
43. Gertraud Maskarinec, James Cooper and Leslie Swygert, 'Investigation of Increased Incidence in Childhood Leukemia Near Radio Towers in

Hawaii: Preliminary Observations', *Journal of Environmental Pathology, Toxicology and Oncology: Official Organ of the International Society for Environmental Toxicology and Cancer* 13, no. 1 (1994): 33–37.

44. Michael Kundi, 'Evidence for Childhood Cancers (Leukemia)', Report for the BioInitiative Working Group, July 2007.

45. Birgitta Floderus et al., 'Occupational Exposure to Electromagnetic Fields in Relation to Leukemia and Brain Tumors: A Case-control Study in Sweden', *Cancer Causes & Control* 4 (1993): 465–476.

46. De-Kun Li, Hong Chen and Roxana Odouli, 'Maternal Exposure to Magnetic Fields During Pregnancy in Relation to the Risk of Asthma in Offspring', *Archives of Pediatrics & Adolescent Medicine* 165, no. 10 (2011): 945–950.

47. G.L. Carlo and T.J. Mariea, 'Wireless Radiation in the Aetiology and Treatment of Autism: Clinical Observations and Mechanisms', *Journal of the Australasian College of Nutritional and Environmental Medicine* 26, no. 2 (2007): 3–7.

48. Robert C. Kane, 'A Possible Association Between Fetal/Neonatal Exposure to Radiofrequency Electromagnetic Radiation and the Increased Incidence of Autism Spectrum Disorders (ASD)', *Medical Hypotheses* 62, no. 2 (2004): 195–197.

49. Martha R. Herbert and Cindy Sage, 'Autism and EMF? Plausibility of a Pathophysiological link–Part I', *Pathophysiology* 20, no. 3 (2013): 191–209.

50. Laura Birks et al., 'Maternal Cell Phone Use During Pregnancy And Child Behavioral Problems in Five Birth Cohorts', *Environment International* 104 (2017): 122–131.

51. 'Wireless and EMF Reduction for Autism', Clear Light Ventures, 31 July 2014, https://www.clearlightventures.com/blog/2014/07/emf-reduction-for-autism.html

52. De-Kun Li et al., 'A Prospective Study of In-utero Exposure to Magnetic Fields and the Risk of Childhood Obesity', *Scientific Reports* 2, no. 1 (2012): 540.

53. Alasdair Philips et al., 'Brain Tumours: Rise in Glioblastoma Multiforme Incidence in England 1995–2015 Suggests an adverse Environmental or Lifestyle Factor', *Journal of Environmental and Public Health* 2018 (2018).

54. Lennart Hardell, Michael Carlberg, and Kjell Hansson Mild, 'Use of Wireless Phones and Evidence for Increased Risk of Brain Tumors',

Pathophysiology 20, no. 2 (2013): 85–110, https://doi.org/10.1016/j.pathophys.2012.11.001; L. Lloyd Morgan et al., 'Mobile Phone Radiation Causes Brain Tumors and Should Be Classified as a Probable Human Carcinogen (2A)', *International Journal of Oncology* 46, no. 5 (2015): 1865–1871; Manya Prasad et al., 'Mobile Phone Use and Risk of Brain Tumours: A Systematic Review of Association Between Study Quality, Source of Funding, and Research Outcomes', *Neurological Sciences* 38 (2017): 797–810; Ming Yang et al., 'Mobile Phone Use and Glioma Risk: A Systematic Review and Meta-analysis', *PloS one* 12, no. 5 (2017): e0175136; Michael Carlberg and Lennart Hardell, 'Pooled Analysis of Swedish Case-control Studies During 1997–2003 and 2007–2009 on Meningioma Risk Associated with the Use of Mobile and Cordless Phones', *Oncology Reports* 33, no. 6 (2015): 3093–3098.

55. Devra Lee Davis et al., 'Swedish Review Strengthens Grounds for Concluding That Radiation from Cellular and Cordless Phones Is a Probable Human Carcinogen', *Pathophysiology* 20, no. 2 (2013): 123-129, https://doi.org/10.1016/j.pathophys.2013.03.001.

56. Siegal Sadetzki et al., 'Cellular Phone Use and Risk of Benign and Malignant Parotid Gland Tumors – A Nationwide Case-control Study', *American Journal of Epidemiology* 167, no. 4 (2008): 457–467.

57. Lönn, Stefan et akl., 'Mobile Phone Use and the Risk of Acoustic Neuroma.' *Epidemiology* (2004): 653–659.

58. Lennart Hardell, Michael Carlberg, and Kjell Hansson Mild. 'Use of Mobile Phones and Cordless Phones is Associated with Increased Risk for Glioma and Acoustic Neuroma', *Pathophysiology* 20, no. 2 (2013): 85–110.

59. CL Sage, 'Evidence for Breast Cancer Promotion (Melatonin Studies in Cells and Animals)', Report for the BioInitiative Working Group, July 2007.

60. Dana P. Loomis, David A. Savitz and Cande V. Ananth, 'Breast cancer Mortality Among Female Electrical Workers in the United States', *JNCI: Journal of the National Cancer Institute* 86, no. 12 (1994): 921–925.

61. Samuel Milham, 'A Cluster of Male Breast Cancer in Office Workers', *American Journal of Industrial Medicine* 46, no. 1 (2004): 86–87.

62. Igor Yakymenko et al., 'Long-term Exposure to Microwave Radiation Provokes Cancer Growth: Evidence from Radars and Mobile Communication Systems', *Experimental Oncology* 33 (2011): 62–70.

63. S. Braune et al., 'Resting Blood Pressure Increase During Exposure to a Radio-frequency Electromagnetic Field', *The Lancet* 351, no. 9119 (1998): 1857–1858.

64. Joseph Mercola, *EMF*D: 5G, Wi-Fi & Cell Phones: Hidden Harms and How to Protect Yourself* (Carlsbad, CA: Hay House, 2020), chapter 5.

65. Martin L. Pall, 'Wi-Fi is An Important Threat to Human Health', *Environmental Research* 164 (2018): 405–416.

66. G. J. Hyland, 'Physics and Biology of Mobile Telephony', *The Lancet* 356, no. 9244 (2000): 1833–1836.

67. B. Stein and Mantle J., *The Microwave Delusion* (Tolworth: Grosvenor House Publishing, 2020), 20.

68. Alexandra Sims, 'Schoolgirl Jenny Fry Found Hanged after "Suffering from Allergy to WiFi"', *Independent*, 1 December 2015.

69. Blank, *Overpowered*, 223–4.

70. Stein and Mantle, *The Microwave Delusion*, 25.

71. William J. Rea et al., 'Electromagnetic Field Sensitivity', *Journal of Bioelectricity* 10, no. 1–2 (1991): 241–256; Olle Johansson, 'Aspects of Studies on the Functional Impairment Electrohypersensitivity', *IOP Conference Series: Earth and Environmental Science* 10, no. 1 (IOP Publishing, 2010): 012005.

72. Igor Belyaev et al., 'EUROPAEM EMF Guideline 2016 for the Prevention, Diagnosis and Treatment of EMF-related Health Problems and Illnesses', *Reviews on Environmental Health* 31, no. 3 (2016): 363–397.

73. Stein and Mantle, *The Microwave Delusion*, 36–39.

74. Erica Mallery-Blythe, '2020 Consensus Statement of UK and International Medical and Scientific Experts and Practitioners on Health Effects of Non-Ionising Radiation (NIR)', PHIRE, 10 November 2020, https://phiremedical.org/wp-content/uploads/2020/11/2020-Non-Ionising-Radiation-Consensus-Statement.pdf.

75. Alison Benjamin, 'Fears for Crops As Shock Figures from America Show Scale of Bee Catastrophe', *Observer*, 2 May 2010.

76. Stefan Kimmel et al., 'Electromagnetic Radiation: Influences on Honeybees (*Apis mellifera*)', *Preprint* (Baden-Baden: IIAS-InterSymp Conference, 2007), 1–6.

77. Ved Parkash Sharma and Neelima R. Kumar, 'Changes in Honeybee Behaviour and Biology Under the Influence of Cellphone Radiations', *Current Science(Bangalore)* 98, no. 10 (2010): 1376–1378.

78. Richard Odemer and Franziska Odemer, 'Effects of Radiofrequency Electromagnetic Radiation (RF-EMF) on Honey Bee Queen Development and Mating Success.' *Science of the Total Environment* 661 (2019): 553–562.

79. Daniel Favre, 'Mobile Phone-induced Honeybee Worker Piping.' *Apidologie* 42, no. 3 (2011): 270–279.
80. S. Sainudeen Sahib, 'Electromagnetic Radiation (EMR) Clashes with Honey Bees.' *International Journal of Environmental Sciences* 1, no. 5 (2011): 897–900.
81. Lukas H. Margaritis et al., 'Drosophila Oogenesis As A Bio-marker Responding to EMF Sources.' *Electromagnetic Biology and Medicine* 33, no. 3 (2014): 165–189.
82. Alain Thill, Marie-Claire Cammaerts and Alfonso Balmori, 'Biological Effects of Electromagnetic Fields on Insects: A Systematic Review and Meta-analysis.' *Reviews on Environmental Health* (2023).
83. Ulrich Warnke, 'Bees, Birds and Mankind: Destroying Nature by "Electrosmog"', *Effects of Wireless Communication Technologies* (Kempten: The Competence Initiative for the Protection of Humanity, Environment and Democracy, 2009).
84. Alfonso Balmori, 'Possible Effects of Electromagnetic Fields from Phone Masts on A Population of White Stork (Ciconia Ciconia).' *Electromagnetic Biology and Medicine* 24, no. 2 (2005): 109–119.
85. Sadequl Islam et al., '4G Mobile Phone Radiation Alters Some Immunogenic and Vascular Gene Expressions, and Gross and Microscopic and Biochemical Parameters in the Chick Embryo Model.' *Veterinary Medicine and Science* 9, no. 6 (2023): 2648–2659.
86. Albert M. Manville, 'Bird Strikes and Electrocutions At Power Lines, Communication Towers, and Wind Turbines: State of the Art and State of the Science – Next Steps Toward Mitigation', *USDA Forest Service General Technical Report PSW-GTR-191* (2005): 1051–1064.
87. Alfonso Balmori, and Örjan Hallberg, 'The Urban Decline of the House Sparrow (Passer domesticus): A Possible Link with Electromagnetic Radiation.' *Electromagnetic Biology and Medicine* 26, no. 2 (2007): 141–151.
88. Joris Everaert and Dirk Bauwens, 'A Possible Effect of Electromagnetic Radiation from Mobile Phone Base Stations on the Number of Breeding House Sparrows (Passer domesticus).' *Electromagnetic Biology and Medicine* 26, no. 1 (2007): 63–72.
89. Alfonso Balmori, 'Mobile Phone Mast Effects on Common Frog (Rana temporaria) Tadpoles: The City Turned into a Laboratory.' *Electromagnetic Biology and Medicine* 29, no. 1–12 (2010): 31–35.

90. E. Malkemper et al., 'Magnetoreception in the Wood Mouse (Apodemus sylvaticus): Influence of Weak Frequency-modulated Radio Frequency Fields.' *Scientific Reports* 5, no. 1 (2015): 9917.

91. *Klaus Heinrich* Vanselow et al, 'Solar Storms May Trigger Sperm Whale Strandings: Explanation Approaches for Multiple Strandings in the North Sea in 2016.' *International Journal of Astrobiology* 17, no. 4 (2018): 336–344.

92. Daniel Nyqvist et al., 'Electric and Magnetic Senses in Marine Animals, and Potential Behavioral Effects of Electromagnetic Surveys.' *Marine Environmental Research* 155 (2020): 104888.

93. Alfonso Balmori-de la Puente, and Alfonso Balmori, 'Potential Effects of Anthropogenic Radiofrequency Radiation on Cetaceans.' *Radiation* 4, no. 1 (2023): 1–16.

94. A.P. Klimley et al., 'A Call to Assess the Impacts of Electromagnetic Fields from Subsea Cables on the Movement Ecology of Marine Migrants', *Conservation Science and Practice* 3, no. 7 (2021): e436, https://doi.org/10.1111/csp2.436.

95. Cornelia Waldmann-Selsam et al., 'Radiofrequency Radiation Injures Trees Around Mobile Phone Base Stations.' *Science of the Total Environment* 572 (2016): 554–569.

96. David Roux et al., 'High Frequency (900 MHz) Low Amplitude (5 V m− 1) electromagnetic Field: A Genuine Environmental Stimulus that Affects Transcription, Translation, Calcium and Energy Charge in Tomato.' *Planta* 227 (2008): 883–891.

97. Edna Ben-Izhak Monselise, Abraham H. Parola and Daniel Kost, 'Low-frequency Electromagnetic Fields Induce A Stress Effect Upon Higher Plants, As Evident By The Universal Stress Signal, Alanine.' *Biochemical and Biophysical Research Communications* 302, no. 2 (2003): 427–434.

98. Mirta Tkalec, Krešimir Malarić and Branka Pevalek-Kozlina, 'Exposure to Radiofrequency Radiation Induces Oxidative Stress in Duckweed Lemna Minor L.' *Science of the Total Environment* 388, no. 1–3 (2007): 78–89.

99. Ved Parkash Sharma et al., 'Cell Phone Radiations Affect Early Growth of *Vigna radiata* (Mung Bean) Through Biochemical Alterations.' *Zeitschrift für Naturforschung C* 65, no. 1–2 (2010): 66–72.

100. Gerhard Soja et al., 'Growth and Yield of Winter Wheat (*Triticum aestivum L.*) and Corn (*Zea mays L.*) Near A High Voltage Transmission Line.' *Bioelectromagnetics* 24, no. 2 (2003): 91–102.

101. '5G: Is It Safe?', PHIRE, 15 June 2022, https://phiremedical.org/5g.
102. ICBE-EMF (International Commission on the Biological Effects of Electromagnetic Fields), 'Scientific Evidence Invalidates Health Assumptions Underlying the FCC and ICNIRP Exposure Limit Determinations for Radiofrequency Radiation: Implications for 5G.' *Environmental Health* 21, no. 1 (2022): 92.
103. Gal Shafirstein, and Eduardo G. Moros, 'Modelling Millimetre Wave Propagation and Absorption in High Resolution Skin Model: The Effect of Sweat Glands.' *Physics in Medicine & Biology* 56, no. 5 (2011): 1329.
104. 'Letter to the FCC from Dr Yael Stein, MD, in Opposition to the 5G Spectrum Frontiers Millimetre Wave Technology', Environmental Health Trust, 9 July 2016, https://ehtrust.org/letter-fcc-dr-yael-stein-md-opposition-5g-spectrum-frontiers.
105. ICBE-EMF, 'Scientific Evidence Invalidates Health Assumptions'.
106. Mercola, *EMF*D*, chapter 2.
107. Mercola, chapter 2.
108. 'Stop 5G on Earth and in Space', 5G Space Appeal, https://www.5gspaceappeal.org/the-appeal.
109. DeBaun, *Radiation Nation*, 43–45.
110. John William Frank, 'Electromagnetic Fields, 5G and Health: What About the Precautionary Principle?.' *Journal of Epidemiology and Community Health* 75 (2021): 562–566.
111. 'Radiofrequency Radiation from Wireless Communications Sources: Are Safety Limits Valid?' An ICBE-EMF Workshop at the Royal Society of Medicine, London, 14 June 2023.
112. Ali Hines, 'Decade of Defiance, Global Witness', 29 September 2022, https://www.globalwitness.org/en/campaigns/environmental-activists/decade-defiance.
113. D. Michaels, *Doubt is Their Product: How Industry's Assault on Science Threatens Your Health* (NY: Oxford University Press, 2008), 79 et seq.
114. DeBaun, Radiation Nation, 133–4; Mercola, *EMF*D*, chapter 3, 59 et seq.
115. ICBE-EMF, 'Scientific Evidence Invalidates Health Assumptions'.
116. Martin L. Pall, 'Microwave Electromagnetic'.
117. ICNIRP Guidelines, 1998.
118. ICBE-EMF, 'Scientific Evidence Invalidates Health Assumptions'.

119. Cindy Sage, and David O. Carpenter, 'Public Health Implications of Wireless Technologies.' *Pathophysiology* 16, no. 2–3 (2009): 233–246.

120. D. Davis, *Disconnect*, 90.

121. J. Wiart et al., 'Analysis of RF Exposure in the Head Tissues of Children and Adults.' *Physics in Medicine & Biology* 53, no. 13 (2008): 3681.

122. Andreas Christ et al., 'Age-dependent Tissue-specific Exposure of Cell Phone Users.' *Physics in Medicine & Biology* 55, no. 7 (2010): 1767.

123. Joseph Wiemels, 'Perspectives on the Causes of Childhood Leukemia.' *Chemico-biological Interactions* 196, no. 3 (2012): 59–67.

124. Paul Ben Ishai et al., 'Problems in Evaluating the Health Impacts of Radio Frequency Radiation.' *Environmental Research* (2023): 115038.

125. Priyanka Bandara and David O. Carpenter, 'Planetary Electromagnetic Pollution: It Is Time To Assess Its Impact.' *The Lancet Planetary Health* 2, no. 12 (2018): e512–e514.

126. Blank, *Overpowered*, 163.

127. Devra Davis et al., 'Wireless Technologies, Non-Ionizing Electromagnetic Fields and Children: Identifying and Reducing Health Risks.' *Current Problems in Pediatric and Adolescent Health Care* (2023): 101374.

128. Igor Belyaev et al., 'EUROPAEM EMF Guideline 2016 for the Prevention, Diagnosis and Treatment of EMF-related Health Problems and Illnesses" *Reviews on Environmental Health*, vol. 31, no. 3, 2016, pp. 363–397. https://doi.org/10.1515/reveh-2016-0011

129. 'Italy Court Ruling Links Mobile Phone Use to Tumor', Reuters, 19 October 2012, https://www.reuters.com/article/idUSBRE89I0V4.

130. Lennart Hardell, 'Long-term Use of Cellular and Cordless Phones and the Risk of Brain Tumours', *Occupational and Environmental Medicine* 64, no.9 (2007): 626–632; ICEMS Position Paper on the Cerebral Tumor Court Case.

131. Reuters, 'Italy Court Ruling'.

Chapter Seven

1. Cother Hajat and Emma Stein, 'The Global Burden of Multiple Chronic Conditions: A Narrative Review', *Preventive Medicine Reports* 12 (2018): 284–293.

2. Janna G. Koppe et al., 'Exposure to Multiple Environmental Agents and Their Effect', *Acta Paediatrica* 95 (2006): 106–113.

3. Øistein Svanes et al., 'Cleaning at Home and at Work In Relation to Lung Function Decline and Airway Obstruction', *American Journal of Respiratory and Critical Care Medicine* 197, no. 9 (2018): 1157–1163.
4. Elissa M. Abrams. 'Cleaning Products and Asthma Risk: a Potentially Important Public Health Concern', *Cmaj* 192, no. 7 (2020): E164–E165.
5. Arezoo Campbell, 'The Potential Role of Aluminium in Alzheimer's Disease', *Nephrology Dialysis Transplantation* 17, no. suppl._2 (2002): 17–20; Matthew Mold, Dorcas Umar, Andrew King and Christopher Exley, 'Aluminium in Brain Tissue in Autism', *Journal of Trace Elements in Medicine and Biology* 46 (2018): 76–82; Philippa D Darbre, Ferdinando Mannello and Christopher Exley, 'Aluminium and Breast Cancer: Sources of Exposure, Tissue Measurements and Mechanisms of Toxicological Actions on Breast Biology', *Journal of Inorganic Biochemistry* 128 (2013): 257–261.
6. E. Horak et al., 'Effects of Nickel Chloride and Nickel Carbonyl upon Glucose Metabolism in Rats', *Annals of Clinical & Laboratory Science* 8, no. 6 (1978): 476–482.
7. Gang Liu et al., 'Nickel Exposure is Associated with the Prevalence of Type 2 diabetes in Chinese Adults.' *International Journal of Epidemiology* 44, no. 1 (2015): 240–248.
8. Tim Smedley, *Clearing the Air: The Beginning and the End of Air Pollution* (London: Bloomsbury Sigma, 2019), footnote 72.
9. Maurício Martins da Silva et al., 'Inhibition of Type 1 Iodothyronine Deiodinase by Bisphenol A', *Hormone and Metabolic Research* 51, no. 10 (2019): 671–677.
10. John L. Wilkinson et al., 'Pharmaceutical Pollution of the World's Rivers.' *Proceedings of the National Academy of Sciences* 119, no. 8 (2022): e2113947119.
11. Muhammad Syafrudin et al., 'Pesticides in Drinking Water – A Review.' *International Journal of Environmental Research and Public Health* 18, no. 2 (2021): 468. s
12. W.W. Nazaroff and C.J. Weschler, 'Cleaning Products and Air Fresheners: Exposure to Primary and Secondary Air Pollutants', *Atmospheric Environment* 38, no. 18 (2004): 2841–2865, https://www.sciencedirect.com/science/article/abs/pii/S1352231004002171.
13. Mohamed I. Hamdouk et al., 'Paraphenylene Diamine Hair Dye Poisoning', in *Clinical Nephrotoxins: Renal Injury from Drugs and Chemicals*, eds. Marc E. Broe, George A. Porter, William M. Bennett and Gert

A. Verpooten (Boston, MA: Springer US, 2008), 871–879; Manuela Gago-Dominguez et al., 'Use of Permanent Hair Dyes and Bladder-cancer Risk', *International Journal of Cancer* 91, no. 4 (2001): 575–579; Sanna Heikkinen et al., 'Does Hair Dye Use Increase the Risk of Breast Cancer? A Population-based Case-Control Study of Finnish Women', *PloS one* 10, no. 8 (2015): e0135190.

14. Che-Jung Chang et al., 'Use of Straighteners and Other Hair Products and Incident Uterine Cancer', *JNCI: Journal of the National Cancer Institute* 114, no. 12 (2022): 1636–1645; Peter F. Infante et al,. 'Vinyl Chloride Propellant in Hair Spray and Angiosarcoma of the Liver Among Hairdressers and Barbers', *International Journal of Occupational and Environmental Health* 15, no. 1 (2009): 36–42.

15. Murali K Matta et al., 'Effect of Sunscreen Application under Maximal Use Conditions on Plasma Concentration of Sunscreen Active Ingredients: A Randomized Clinical Trial', *Jama* 321, no. 21 (2019): 2082–2091; Antonia M Calafat et al., 'Concentrations of the Sunscreen Agent Benzophenone-3 in Residents of the United States: National Health and Nutrition Examination Survey 2003–2004', *Environmental health Perspectives* 116, no. 7 (2008): 893–897.

16. Zoe Diana Draelos, 'Are Sunscreens Safe?' *Journal of Cosmetic Dermatology* 9, no. 1 (2010): 1–2.

17. Campbell, 'The Potential Role of Aluminium in Alzheimer's Disease', 17–20; Mold, Umar, King and Exley, 'Aluminium in Brain Tissue in Autism', 76–82; Darbre, Mannello and Exley, 'Aluminium and Breast Cancer', 257–261.

18. Environmental Working Group, 2012, 'The Scent of Danger: Are There Toxic Ingredients in Perfumes and Colognes?' *Scientific American*, 29 September 2012, https://www.scientificamerican.com/article/toxic-perfumes-and-colognes.

19. Lareina Wujanto, and Sarah Wakelin, 'Allergic Contact Dermatitis to Colophonium in a Sanitary pad – an Overlooked Allergen?.' *Contact Dermatitis* 66, no. 3 (2012): 161–162.

20. N. Hill et al., 'Single Blind, Randomised, Comparative Study of the Bug Buster Kit and Over The Counter Pediculicide Treatments Against Head Lice in the United Kingdom.' *British Medical Journal* 331, no. 7513 (2005): 384–387.

21. My thanks to holistic vet, Richard Allport, for this tip.

22. Kira Oz, Bareket Merav, Sabach Sara and Dubowski Yael, 'Volatile Organic Compound Emissions from Polyurethane Mattresses Under Variable Environmental Conditions', *Environmental Science & Technology* 53, no. 15 (2019): 9171–9180; E.M. Beckett et al., 'Evaluation of Volatile Organic Compound (VOC) Emissions from Memory Foam Mattresses and Potential Implications for Consumer Health Risk', *Chemosphere* 303 (2022): 134945.

23. National Toxicology Program, 'Report on Carcinogens, 14th edition: 1,4-dichlorobenzene', Report on Carcinogens, 14th ed. (Research Triangle Park, NC: U.S. Department of Health and Human Services, 2016), 139–141; James A. Barter and James H. Sherman, 'An Evaluation of the Carcinogenic Hazard of 1,4-Dichlorobenzene Based on Internationally Recognized Criteria', Regulatory Toxicology and Pharmacology 29, no.1 (1999), 64–79, https://doi.org/10.1006/rtph.1998.1269.

24. Jane Caldwell, Ruth Lunn and Avima Ruder, 'Tetrachloroethylene (perc, tetra, PCE)', *IARC Monographs on the Evaluation of Carcinogenic Risks to Humans* 63 (1995): 159–221.

25. Peter B. Bethwaite, Neil Pearce and James Fraser, 'Cancer Risks in Painters: Study Based on the New Zealand Cancer Registry,' *British Journal of Industrial Medicine* 47, no. 11 (1990): 742.

Conclusion

1. An excellent example is 'Poisoned Planet: How Constant Exposure to Man-made Chemicals is putting Your Life At Risk', 2014, by Julian Cribb, an Australian journalist. My thanks to Dr Shideh Pouria for gifting me a copy; it made the process of writing this book feel a little less lonely.

2. Rafia Farooq Peer and Nadeem Shabir, 'Iatrogenesis: A Review on Nature, Extent, and Distribution of healthcare Hazards.' *Journal of Family Medicine and Primary Care* 7, no. 2 (2018): 309.

3. Robin Wall Kimmerer, *Braiding Sweetgrass* (Penguin/Random House, UK, 2013), 195.

Appendix I

1. Michaela Roberts et al., 'The Contribution of Environmental Science to Mental Health Research: A Scoping Review.' *International Journal of Environmental Research and Public Health* 20, no. 7 (2023): 5278.

2. Philippe Grandjean and Philip J. Landrigan, 'Neurobehavioural Effects of Developmental Toxicity.' *The Lancet Neurology* 13, no. 3 (2014): 330–338.

3. Lilian Calderón-Garcidueñas et al., 'Air Pollution, Combustion and Friction Derived Nanoparticles, and Alzheimer's Disease in Urban Children and Young Adults.' *Journal of Alzheimer's Disease* 70, no. 2 (2019): 343–360.

4. Sonali Bose et al., 'Prenatal Particulate Air Pollution Exposure and Sleep Disruption in Preschoolers: Windows of Susceptibility.' *Environment International* 124 (2019): 329–335.

5. Marie-Claire Flores-Pajot et al., 'Childhood Autism Spectrum Disorders and Exposure to Nitrogen Dioxide, and Particulate Matter Air Pollution: A Review and Meta-analysis.' *Environmental Research* 151 (2016): 763–776.

6. Ioannis Bakolis et al., 'Mental Health Consequences of Urban Air Pollution: Prospective Population-based Longitudinal Survey.' *Social Psychiatry and Psychiatric Epidemiology* 56 (2021): 1587–1599.

7. Xuelin Gu et al., 'Association Between Particulate Matter Air Pollution and Risk of Depression and Suicide: Systematic Review and Meta-analysis-RETRACTION.' *The British Journal of Psychiatry* 217, no. 2 (2020): 459–459.

8. P.C. Bello-Medina, E. Rodríguez-Martínez, R.A. Prado-Alcalá and S. Rivas-Arancibia, 'Ozone Pollution, Oxidative Stress, Synaptic Plasticity, and Neurodegeneration.' *Neurología (English Edition)* 37, no. 4 (2022): 277–286.

9. Amy Ronaldson et al., 'Associations Between Air Pollution and Mental Health Service Use in Dementia: A Retrospective Cohort Study', *BMJ Mental Health* 26, no. 1 (2023).

10. Edmond D. Shenassa et al., 'Dampness and Mold in the Home and Depression: An Examination of Mold-related Illness and Perceived Control of One's Home as Possible Depression Pathways.' *American Journal of Public Health* 97, no. 10 (2007): 1893–1899.

11. Mary Ackerley, 'Brain on Fire: The Role of Mold in Triggering Psychiatric Symptoms', Paradigm Change, 1 May 2015, https://irp-cdn.multiscreensite.com/562d25c6/files/uploaded/Brain-on-Fire-article-by-Dr-Mary-Ackerley_2014.pdf.

12. Cort Johnson, 'Brains on Fire, Swollen Brains, Toxins and Neuroinflammation – by Dr. Mary Ackerley', Health Rising, 30 December 2019, https://www.healthrising.org/blog/2019/12/30/brains-on-fire-swollen-brains-toxins-and-neuroinflammation-by-mary-dr-ackerley.

INDEX

ABOUT THE AUTHOR

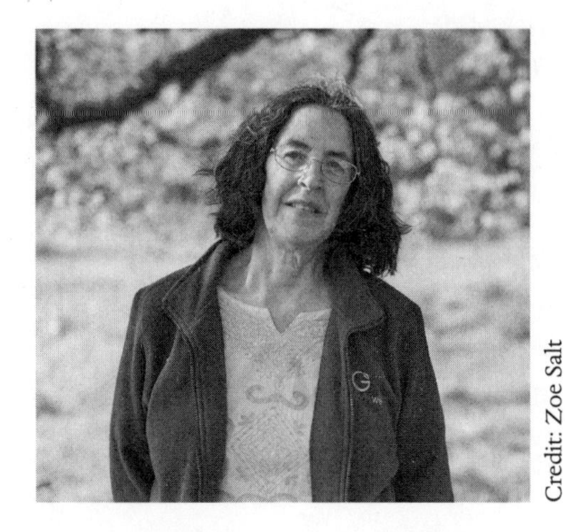

Credit: Zoe Salt

Jenny Goodman is a medical doctor, lecturer and broadcaster. She qualified at Leeds University School of Medicine and worked as a junior doctor but, disillusioned with conventional medicine's inability to heal sick people and its failure to enquire about the causes of illness or to do preventive healthcare, she went on to study ecological medicine with the British Society for Ecological Medicine (BSEM). The BSEM is a group of doctors and other practitioners who help patients to attain dramatically better health through changes in diet and nutrition, and through detoxification.

Jenny has been practising ecological medicine for twenty-two years and is the author of *Staying Alive in Toxic Times*. She appeared with Terry Pratchett in ITV's documentary *What's in Your Mouth?* and has been featured on the Victoria Derbyshire show, BBC One's *Inside Out* and numerous other TV and radio shows.